TRAUMATIC DENTAL INJURIES
– A Manual

Third Edition

J. O. ANDREASEN

L. K. BAKLAND

M. T. FLORES

F. M. ANDREASEN

L. ANDERSSON

⟨W⟩WILEY-BLACKWELL

This edition first published 2011
© 1999 Munksgaard
© 2003 Blackwell Munksgaard
© 2011 J.O. Andreasen, L.K. Bakland, M.T. Flores, F.M. Andreasen and L. Andersson

Blackwell Publishing was acquired by John Wiley & Sons in February 2007. Blackwell's publishing programme has been merged with Wiley's global Scientific, Technical, and Medical business to form Wiley-Blackwell.

Registered office
John Wiley & Sons Ltd, The Atrium, Southern Gate, Chichester, West Sussex, PO19 8SQ, United Kingdom

Editorial offices
9600 Garsington Road, Oxford, OX4 2DQ, United Kingdom
The Atrium, Southern Gate, Chichester, West Sussex, PO19 8SQ, United Kingdom
2121 State Avenue, Ames, Iowa 50014-8300, USA

First edition published 1999
Second edition 2003
Third edition 2011

For details of our global editorial offices, for customer services and for information about how to apply for permission to reuse the copyright material in this book please see our website at www.wiley.com/wiley-blackwell.

Library of Congress Cataloging-in-Publication Data
Traumatic dental injuries : a manual / J.O. Andreasen ... [et al.]. – 3rd ed.
        p. ; cm.
    Includes bibliographical references and index.
    ISBN 978-1-4051-9061-9 (pbk. : alk. paper)   1. Teeth–Wounds and injuries–Handbooks, manuals, etc.   2. Dentistry, Operative–Handbooks, manuals,
etc.   I. Andreasen, J. O.
    [DNLM: 1. Tooth Injuries–diagnosis–Handbooks.   2. Tooth Injuries–therapy–Handbooks. WU 49]
    RK501.5.T73 2011
    617.6044–dc22

                                                                                                                            2010040958

A catalogue record for this book is available from the British Library.

Artwork by Henning Dalhoff Aps, Tue Frigaard Hansen from 360 Degree, Karina Nekes Suhr and Søren Ahrensburg Steno Christensen

Layout by Tue Frigaard Hansen from 360 Degree, Karina Nekes Suhr and Søren Ahrensburg Steno Christensen

Set in 9/12 pt Helvetica by Toppan Best-set Premedia Limited
Printed in Singapore

1   2011

Preface to Third Edition

The third edition of *Traumatic Dental Injuries – A Manual* includes several new aspects of dental traumatology and an updating of existing material. The new sections that have been included describe soft tissue injuries associated with dental trauma, show how decoronation of ankylosed anterior teeth in adolescents can preserve the alveolar process for later implant placement or prosthodontic restoration and identify predictors for pulpal and periodontal ligament healing complications as well as for tooth loss. Furthermore the use of an internet-based interactive *Dental Trauma Guide* to predict healing complication for individual trauma scenarios is introduced. An added bonus is an enclosed DVD that shows animated treatment procedures for all trauma entities.

J. O. Andreasen, L. K. Bakland, M. T. Flores, F. M. Andreasen, L. Andersson
Copenhagen, January 2011

Preface to Second Edition

In this second edition, the epidemiological section on global trauma frequencies has been updated and all chapters have been revised, especially with respect to the urgency of acute treatment. Furthermore, the chapter on prevention of oral injuries has been expanded. New chapters include diagnosis of pulp and periodontal healing complications, long-term prognosis of the various trauma entities, and information to the patient subsequent to emergency treatment. Finally, a chapter has been included which deals with the principles of endodontic treatment of traumatized teeth.

J. O. Andreasen, F. M. Andreasen, L. K. Bakland, M. T. Flores
Copenhagen, January 2003

Preface to First Edition

In *Traumatic Dental Injuries – A Manual*, we present the highlights of dental traumatology in a format which will be a ready reference for general practitioners and aid dental students in their studies. Each chapter is designed to describe the principles in the diagnosis and treatment of the specific traumatic dental injury, including treatment objectives, treatment parameters and long-term expectations based on existing long-term studies of various trauma entities. In order to standardize diagnostic and treatment procedures, examination forms and follow-up protocol are provided in the appendices. As no type of dental trauma is 'perfect', a given injury type has been generated electronically by a medical artist, in order to enhance similarities and differences between the various injury groups. Periodontal and pulpal healing for the given injuries are based on recent long-term follow-up studies.

Finally, information to the public is also presented. As the best treatment result follows prompt emergency care, informed individuals at the scene of the injury can aid the dental practitioner in optimizing treatment and hopefully in preventing injuries.

It is the authors' hope that *Traumatic Dental Injuries – A Manual* will fill the gap in dental education and give dental trauma its full birthright.

J. O. Andreasen, F. M. Andreasen, L. K. Bakland, M. T. Flores
Copenhagen, January 1999

Contributors

JENS O. ANDREASEN, DDS, ODONT DR. HC, FRCS
Department of Oral and Maxillofacial Surgery
University Hospital (Rigshospitalet)
Copenhagen
Denmark

LEIF K. BAKLAND, DDS
Diplomate, American Board of Endodontics
Ronald E. Buell Professor of Endodontics
School of Dentistry, Loma Linda University
Loma Linda, California
USA

MARIA T. FLORES, DDS
Professor of Pediatric Dentistry
Faculty of Dentistry
University of Valparaiso
Valparaiso
Chile

FRANCES M. ANDREASEN, DDS, DR. ODONT
Research Associate
Department of Oral and Maxillofacial Surgery
University Hospital (Rigshospitalet)
Copenhagen
Denmark

LARS ANDERSSON, DDS, ODONT DR.
Professor of Oral and Maxillofacial Surgery
Faculty of Dentistry
Kuwait University
Kuwait City
Kuwait

Contents

Epidemiology of Traumatic Dental Injuries

┌─ OBJECTIVES ───┐
│ **1**   Recognize trauma incidence and prevalence in the primary and permanent dentitions. │
│ **2**   Recognize peak incidences of trauma in relation to age and sex.   │
│ **3**   Recognize typical causes of trauma.   │
└──┘

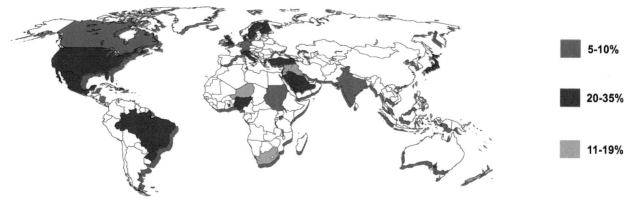

TRAUMA PREVALENCE

The prevalence (i.e. the number of injuries up to a given age) of traumatic dental injuries has been examined in many countries, usually reporting very high figures. [1] It should, however, be noted that most of these studies represent prevalences in various age groups, and therefore these prevalences cannot be compared. When prevalences are specified for 5- and 12-year-olds, the figures can be seen in the maps below. Please note that only countries where reliable figures were available have been included and color-coded.

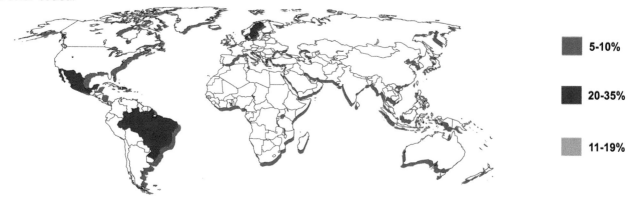

TRAUMA PREVALENCE IN 5-YEAR-OLD CHILDREN

In 5-year-old children, approximately one-third have suffered a traumatic dental injury involving primary teeth, most often tooth luxation; boys have a slightly higher frequency than girls. [1,2]

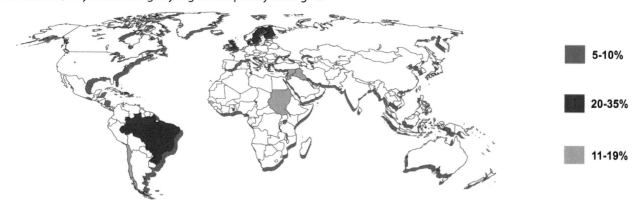

TRAUMA PREVALENCE IN 12-YEAR-OLD CHILDREN

In 12-year-old children, 20–30% of them have suffered dental injuries, with boys' injuries occurring approximately one-third more frequently than girls'. The typical injury is an uncomplicated crown fracture. [1,2]

Traumatic Dental Injuries: A Manual, Third Edition   © J.O. Andreasen, L.K. Bakland, M.T. Flores, F.M. Andreasen and L. Andersson
Published 2011 by Blackwell Publishing Ltd

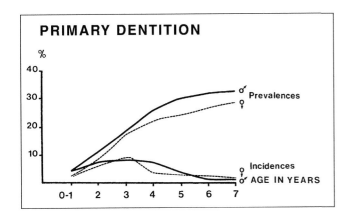

TRAUMA PREVALENCE AND INCIDENCES IN THE PRIMARY DENTITION

Annual trauma incidences (i.e. the number of new injuries occurring during a year) peak in the primary dentition at 2–3 years of age, when motor coordination is developing and the children start moving around on their own. [1,2]

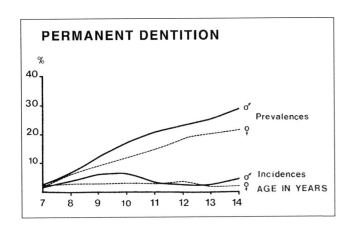

TRAUMA PREVALENCE AND INCIDENCES IN THE PERMANENT DENTITION

In the permanent dentition, peak incidence for boys is found at 9–10 years, during which time vigorous playing and sports activities become more frequent. [1,2]

Longitudinal studies during one year have shown incidences between 1.3 and 4% for school children and 0.4% for all ages in the population of a society.[1]

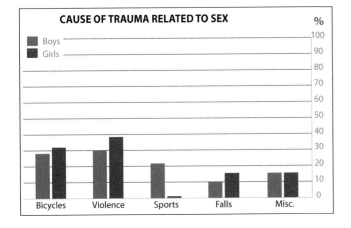

ETIOLOGY OF TRAUMA

The most common causes of injuries in the permanent dentition are falls, followed by traffic injuries, acts of violence and sports accidents.[3]

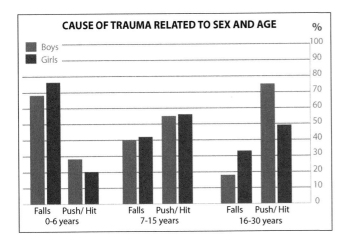

ETIOLOGY OF TRAUMA IN VARIOUS AGE GROUPS

In preschool children (0–6 years) the injuries mainly result from falling and usually occur in the home environment during day time.

In school children (7–15 years) the injuries mainly result from being pushed and hit, and from falling; these occur mainly in school or sports areas during day time.

In adolescents and adults the injuries mainly result from push/hit injuries which predominantly occur during leisure hours.[4]

Pathophysiology and Consequences of Dental Trauma

OBJECTIVES

1 Describe the pathophysiology and effect of trauma.

2 Describe healing events after uncomplicated (separation) injuries to the pulp and periodontium.

3 Describe healing events after complicated (crushing) injuries to the pulp and periodontium.

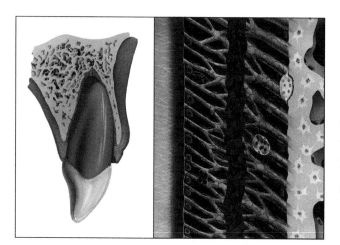

PATHOPHYSIOLOGY OF TRAUMA: SEPARATION INJURY

A traumatic dental injury represents acute transmission of energy to a tooth and its supporting structures, which results in fracture and/or displacement of the tooth and/or separation or crushing of the supporting tissues (gingival, periodontal ligament [PDL] and bone).[5,6] In cases of separation injury (e.g. extrusive luxation), the major part of the injury to the supporting tissues consists of cleavage of intercellular structures (collagen and intercellular substance), with limited damage to the cells in the area of trauma. This implies that wound healing can arise from existing cellular systems with minimal delay.

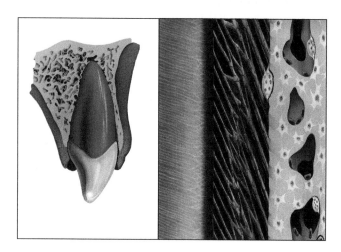

PATHOPHYSIOLOGY OF TRAUMA: CRUSHING INJURY

In contrast to separation injury, in a crushing injury (e.g. lateral luxation and intrusive luxation), there is extensive damage to both cellular and intercellular systems; consequently, damaged tissue must be removed by macrophages and/or osteoclasts before the traumatized tissue can be repaired. In this type of injury, several weeks are added to the healing process and this is reflected in the recommended splinting period.

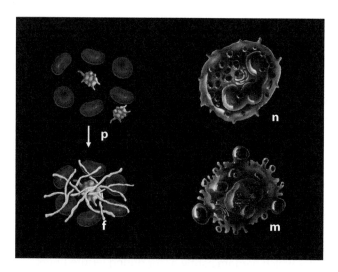

EARLY WOUND HEALING EVENTS

The immediate events following trauma include bleeding from ruptured vessels followed by coagulation.[5,6] In the Figure, components of the pathophysiologic response are described. Platelets (p) in the coagulum play a significant role, not only in transformation of fibrinogen to fibrin (f), but also due to their content of growth factors (e.g. platelet-derived growth factor [PGDF] and transforming growth factors [TGF]-β), which initiate the wound healing process. Thereafter, an influx of neutrophilic leukocytes (n) and macrophages (m) occurs. The first cell type is concerned with infection, while the latter clean the area of damaged tissue and foreign bodies, assisting the neutrophilic leukocytes in defending against or combating microbial colonization, and finally in taking over the platelets' role in directing wound healing events.[5,6]

Traumatic Dental Injuries: A Manual, Third Edition   © J.O. Andreasen, L.K. Bakland, M.T. Flores, F.M. Andreasen and L. Andersson
Published 2011 by Blackwell Publishing Ltd

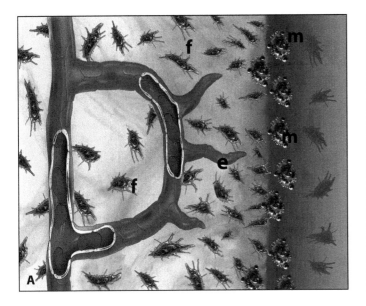

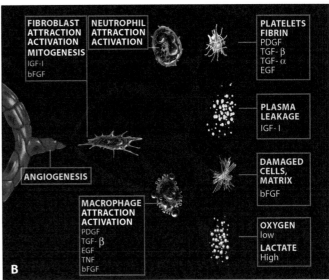

LATER WOUND HEALING EVENTS

Wound healing events comprise revascularization of ischemic tissue and formation of new tissue in case of tissue loss (Figure A). In both instances, wound healing takes place by a coordinated movement of cells into the traumatized area, where macrophages (m) form the healing front, followed by endothelial cells (e) and fibroblasts (f). Vascular loops are formed in a stroma of tissue dominated by immature collagen (Type III) and proliferating fibroblasts. These cells are synchronized via chemical signals released by the involved cells and the surrounding tissue.[5] This phenomenon has been termed the wound healing module (Figure B), and appears to advance in the pulp and periodontium with a speed of approximately 0.5 mm a day.[6]

Below, wound-healing responses will be described as they appear in cases of uncomplicated luxation injuries, with only separation injuries of the PDL and the pulp, and complicated luxation injuries with crushing injuries.[6]

The few experiments carried out on *uncomplicated luxation injuries* indicate the following about the type and chronology of healing:

PDL: After 1 week, new collagen formation starts to unite the severed PDL fibers which leads to initial consolidation of a luxated or a replanted tooth. After 2 weeks, repair of the principal fibers is so advanced that approximately two-thirds of the mechanical strength of the PDL has been restored.[6]

Pulp: In luxated teeth with a severed vascular supply, ingrowth of new vessels into the pulp starts 4 days after injury and proceeds with a speed of approximately 0.5 mm per day in teeth with open apices. Revascularization is markedly influenced by the size of the pulpo-periodontal interface (i.e. diameter of the apical foramen), being complete and predictable in teeth with open apices (≥1.0 mm), and rare in teeth with a narrow apical foramen (<0.5 mm).[6]

The most significant factor that can arrest the revascularization process appears to be colonization of bacteria in the ischemic pulp tissue. The origin of these bacteria can be invasion from dentinal tubules via a crown fracture, or invasion along the blood clot in a severed PDL. Finally, bacteria can be carried to the area via the blood stream (anachoresis). Thus, it has been found that the revascularization process with its endothelial sprouts is often incontinent, allowing corpuscular elements, like erythrocytes and bacteria, to leave the blood stream.[6]

In *complicated luxation injuries*, with *crushing or other damage of the PDL* (e.g. desiccation after avulsion), complicating sequelae may occur which result in root resorption.[6] These processes occur due to the loss of the protecting cementoblast layer and the epithelial rests of Malassez along the root surface, caused by the traumatic events. When these cell layers disappear, there is free access for osteoclasts and macrophages to remove damaged PDL and cementum on the root surface.

Further events are subsequently determined by three factors:

- Eventual exposure of dentinal tubules.
- Content of the pulp, whether it is ischemic and sterile or necrotic and infected.
- Presence of adjacent vital cementoblasts.

The combination of these factors may lead to the healing complications shown on the following pages as the wound healing module involves the injury site.[6-8]

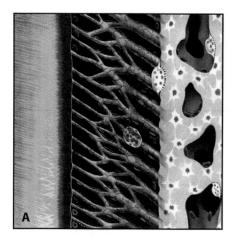
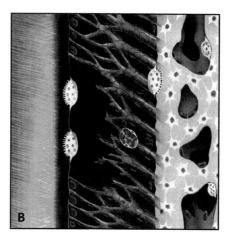
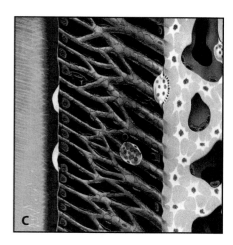

REPAIR-RELATED (SURFACE) RESORPTION

In cases of damage to the layer of the PDL closest to cementum (Figure A), the site will be resorbed by macrophages and osteoclasts, and results in a saucer-shaped cavity on the root surface (Figure B). If this cavity is not in contact with dentinal tubules and the adjacent cementoblast layer is intact, this resorption cavity is repaired by new cementum and insertion of new Sharpey's fibers (Figure C). The ligament width is normal and follows the contours of the defect.[7,8]

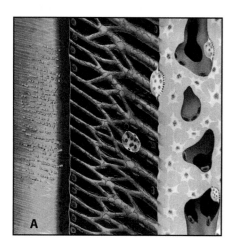
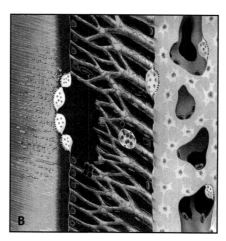
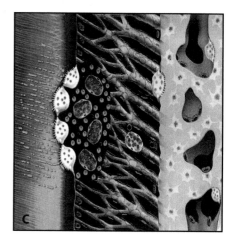

INFECTION-RELATED (INFLAMMATORY) RESORPTION

In the event that the initial resorption penetrates the cementum and exposes dentinal tubules (Figures A and B), toxins from bacteria present in the dentinal tubules and/or the infected root canal can diffuse via the exposed tubules to the PDL. This results in continuation of the osteoclastic process and an associated inflammation in the PDL leading to resorption of the lamina dura and adjacent bone (Figure B) along with resorption of tooth structure. This process is usually progressive until the root canal is exposed. If bacteria are eliminated from the root canal and/or dentinal tubules by proper endodontic therapy, the resorptive process will be arrested. The resorption cavity will then be filled in with cementum (Figure C) or bone, according to the type of vital tissue found next to the resorption site (PDL or bone marrow-derived tissue).[7,8]

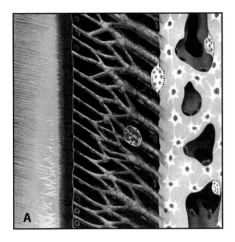
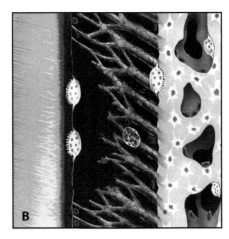
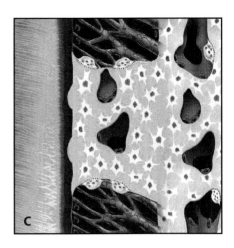

ANKYLOSIS-RELATED (REPLACEMENT) RESORPTION

In cases of extensive damage to the innermost layer of the PDL, competitive healing events will take place whereby healing from the socket wall (creating bone via bone marrow-derived cells) and healing from adjacent PDL next to the root surface (creating cementum and Sharpey's fibers) will take place simultaneously.[7,8]

With cases of moderate injuries (1–4 mm^2), an initial ankylosis is formed (Figures A–C). This can later be replaced with new cementum and PDL, if allowed functional mobility by the use of a semi-rigid splint, or no splinting (transient ankylosis). In this way resorption of the initial ankylosis site may occur.[7]

With larger injuries (>4 mm^2) transient or progressive ankylosis occurs. This leads to the tooth becoming an integral part of the bone remodeling system. The entire process includes osteoclastic resorption dependent on bone remodeling processes, parathyroid hormone-induced resorption, remodeling due to function and resorption due to bacteria present in the gingival area and/or the root canal. All of these processes are very active in children and lead to gradual infraocclusion and arrested development of the alveolar process. In children, this combination of resorption processes leads to loss of ankylosed teeth within 1–5 years. In older individuals, replacement resorption is significantly slower and often allows the tooth to function for longer periods of time (i.e. 5–20 years).

TRANSIENT MARGINAL AND APICAL BREAKDOWN OF BONE

In situations where compression of the PDL has occurred (e.g. lateral luxation and intrusion), macrophage/osteoclast removal of traumatized tissue prior to periodontal healing often results in a *transient marginal breakdown* that is manifested by formation of gingival granulation tissue at the site of compression and a transient radiographic breakdown of the lamina dura at the site involved. After 2–3 months the periodontium will usually be reformed. Likewise, in the apical region a *transient apical breakdown* may occur in teeth with closed apices in cases where pulp healing takes place after luxation injuries (i.e. extrusion, lateral luxation). In these instances a transient radiographic radiolucency is seen as a response to ingrowth of new tissue into the pulp canal (see page 23).[7,8]

PERMANENT MARGINAL BREAKDOWN

The causes of permanent marginal breakdown are the same as described for transient marginal breakdown. However, possibly due to infection or the size of the initial damage, healing does not take place. In some cases bone sequestration may occur. Permanent marginal breakdown may be seen after lateral luxations, avulsion, intrusion, alveolar fracture and jaw fractures.

EFFECT OF TREATMENT ON WOUND HEALING AFTER LUXATION AND REPLANTATION AFTER AVULSION

The value of treatment procedures, such as repositioning and splinting, has not yet been adequately investigated. Evidence to date is discussed in the following sections.

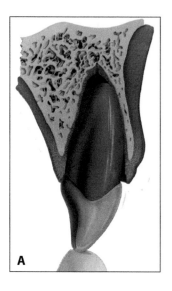 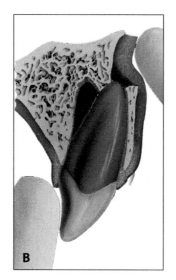 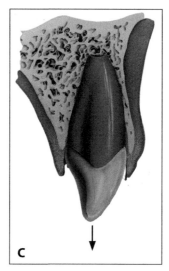 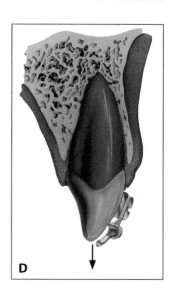

EFFECT OF REPOSITIONING

Depending on the force needed to reposition a displaced tooth, major or minor additional trauma will be transmitted to the periodontium and the pulp. Aside from the need for repositioning with respect to occlusion and esthetics, this negative effect should be assessed in the light of possible benefits in subsequent wound healing with approximation of wound surfaces. In the following, an outline is presented of the known effects of repositioning upon pulpal and periodontal wound healing.

PDL. Incomplete – in contrast to complete – repositioning leads to a slight delay (approximately 2 weeks) in wound healing.[6–8] However, the end result for the PDL is the same. If part of the root surface is exposed to saliva (e.g. extrusive luxation), a loss of attachment in that particular region will occur unless complete repositioning is performed (Figure A). In lateral luxation, the value of repositioning is not known (Figure B). Especially in those cases where forceful repositioning would be necessary, spontaneous readjustment (in young individuals) or orthodontic readjustment should be considered. Occlusal and/or esthetic demands, however, usually require immediate repositioning even in these cases.

After intrusion of permanent teeth, spontaneous re-eruption can usually only be expected in teeth with incomplete root formation (Figure C). In teeth with completed root formation, orthodontic repositioning is probably to be preferred over immediate (surgical) repositioning (after the age of 15 years) in order to enhance marginal bone healing (Figure D). However, there is little definite information available concerning this issue.

Pulp. Optimal repositioning leads to a more rapid and predictable pulpal revascularization.[6–8] Furthermore, if root formation is not complete, there is a good chance of survival of the epithelial root sheath and thereby an optimal chance of continued root growth.

In root fractures, optimal repositioning appears to favor interfragment healing with hard tissue (dentin and cementum) and lessen the chance of pulp necrosis.[9]

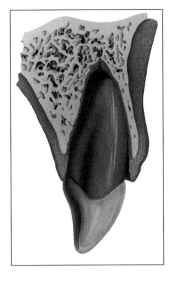
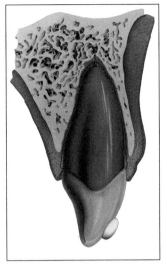

EFFECT OF SPLINTING

PDL. With an uncomplicated rupture of the PDL (e.g. extrusive luxation), rigid splinting does not promote healing.[10] *Flexible splinting* is presently thought to assist periodontal healing, possibly due to more optimal circulatory conditions in PDL, but this effect has not been definitively demonstrated. In situations with massive PDL cell death (e.g. avulsions), prolonged rigid splinting apparently seems to lead to maintenance of initially formed ankylosis sites along the root surface. In these cases, short-term semi-rigid splinting (i.e. 1–2 weeks to permit initial endodontics) appears to be the treatment of choice. Splinting procedures are discussed later (see page 62).

Pulp. Rigid splinting appears to slow down pulpal revascularization.[6] Non-splinting or flexible splinting is to be preferred (see page 62).

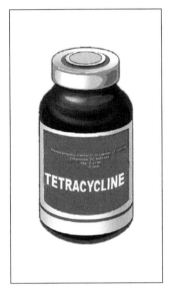
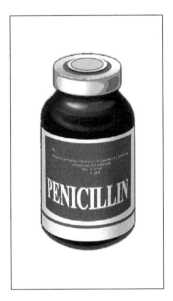

EFFECT OF ANTIBIOTICS

PDL. Under experimental conditions, antibiotics administered either topically for 5 min before replantation of teeth in monkeys or systemically on the day of replantation have been found to decrease the extent of external root resorption.[11-14] The explanation for this is most likely the killing of bacteria on the root surface that otherwise must be eliminated by an inflammatory response, perhaps leading to an osteoclastic attack on the root surface (see page 12).

Pulp. The effect of antibiotics on pulpal healing is yet to be determined. *Systemic* administration of antibiotics after luxations, root fractures and alveolar fractures has not been found in clinical studies to enhance pulpal healing[15]; nor could any effect be seen experimentally after replantation of extracted teeth in monkeys.[12] However, experimental studies in monkeys has shown that a 5-min *topical* application of antibiotics (doxycycline, 1 mg in 20 ml physiologic saline) was found to favor the likelihood of revascularization after replantation of extracted teeth with immature root formation.[11,16]

NOTES

_____

_____

_____

_____

_____

_____

_____

_____

_____

_____

_____

Classification of Dental Injuries

OBJECTIVE

1   Recognize injuries involving the various parts of the tooth and supporting structures.

Dental injuries have been classified according to a variety of factors, such as etiology, anatomy, pathology, or therapeutic considerations.[17,18] The present classification is based on a system adopted by the World Health Organization (WHO) in its *Application of International Classification of Diseases to Dentistry and Stomatology*.[19] However, for the sake of completeness, it has been necessary to define and classify certain trauma entities that were not included in the WHO system. The following classification includes injuries to the teeth, supporting structures, gingiva and oral mucosa and is based on anatomical, therapeutic and prognostic considerations. This classification can be applied to both the permanent and the primary dentitions. The code number is according to the International Classification of Diseases (1995).[19]

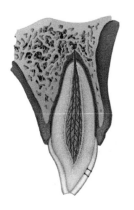
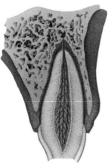
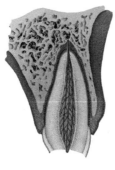

INJURIES TO THE HARD DENTAL TISSUES AND THE PULP

Enamel infraction (S 02.50). An incomplete fracture (crack) of the enamel without loss of tooth structure.

Enamel fracture (uncomplicated crown fracture) (S 02.50). A fracture confined to the enamel with loss of tooth structure.

Enamel–dentin fracture (uncomplicated crown fracture) (S 02.51). A fracture confined to enamel and dentin with loss of tooth structure.

Enamel-dentine-pulp-fracture (S 02.52). A fracture involving enamel and dentin with loss of tooth structure and exposure of the pulp.

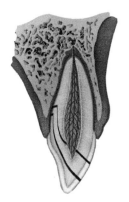
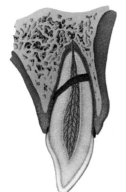
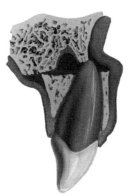

INJURIES TO THE HARD DENTAL TISSUES: THE PULP, PERIODONTAL LIGAMENT AND ALVEOLAR PROCESS

Crown-root fracture (S 02.54). A fracture involving enamel, dentin and cementum. It may or may not expose the pulp.

Root fracture (S 02.53). A fracture involving dentin, cementum and the pulp. Root fractures can be further classified according to displacement of the coronal fragment (see luxation injuries).

Fracture of the mandibular (S 02.60) or **maxillary** (S 02.40) **alveolar socket wall**. A fracture of the alveolar process which involves the alveolar socket (see lateral luxation).

Fracture of the mandibular (S 02.60) or **maxillary** (S 02.40) **alveolar process**. A fracture of the alveolar process that may or may not involve the alveolar socket.

Traumatic Dental Injuries: A Manual, Third Edition   © J.O. Andreasen, L.K. Bakland, M.T. Flores, F.M. Andreasen and L. Andersson
Published 2011 by Blackwell Publishing Ltd

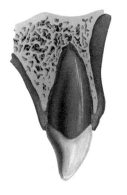
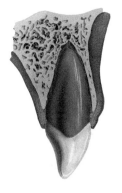
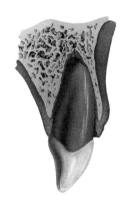

INJURIES TO THE SUPPORTING TISSUES

Concussion (S 03.20). An injury to the tooth-supporting structures without abnormal loosening or displacement of the tooth, but with marked pain to percussion.

Subluxation (loosening) (S 03.20). An injury to the tooth-supporting structures resulting in increased mobility, but without displacement of the tooth.

Extrusive luxation (peripheral dislocation, partial avulsion) (S 03.21). Partial displacement of the tooth out of its socket.

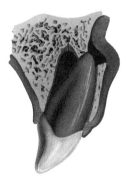
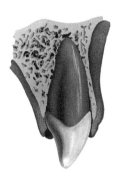
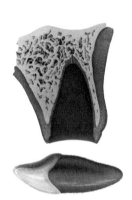

INJURIES TO THE SUPPORTING TISSUES

Lateral luxation (S 03.20). Displacement of the tooth in a direction other than axially. Displacement is accompanied by comminution or fracture of either the labial or the palatal/lingual alveolar bone.

Intrusive luxation (central dislocation) (S 03.21). Displacement of the tooth into the alveolar bone. This injury is accompanied by comminution or fracture of the alveolar socket.

Avulsion (exarticulation) (S 03.22). The tooth is completely displaced out of its socket.

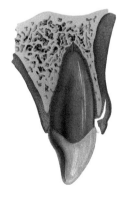
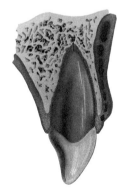
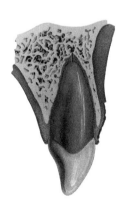

INJURIES TO GINGIVA, ORAL MUCOSA OR SKIN

Abrasion (S01.50). A superficial wound produced by rubbing or scraping of the skin or mucosa leaving a raw, bleeding surface.

Contusion (S01.50). A bruise without a break in the skin or mucosa. Subcutaneous or submucosal hemorrhage in the tissue. A contusion may be isolated to the soft tissue but may also indicate an underlying bone fracture.

Laceration (S01.50). A shallow or deep wound penetrating into the soft tissue, usually produced by a sharp object. May disrupt blood vessels, nerves, muscles and involve salivary glands. Most frequently seen in lips, oral mucosa and gingiva. More seldom the tongue is involved.

Soft tissue avulsion (S01.50). Avulsion (loss of tissue) injuries are rare but seen with bite injuries or as a result of a very deep and extended abrasion.

Examination and Diagnosis

In order to arrive at a timely and accurate diagnosis and the probable extent of injury to the pulp, periodontium and associated structures, a systematic examination of the traumatized patient is essential (see also Appendices 1–3).[20–22] When the patient arrives for treatment of an acute trauma, the oral region is usually heavily contaminated. The first step in the examination procedure, therefore, is to wash the patient's face and oral cavity. If there are soft tissue wounds, a mild detergent should be used. While this is being done, it is possible to get an initial impression of the extent of injury. Thereafter, a series of questions must be asked to aid in diagnosis and treatment planning. These questions include the following.

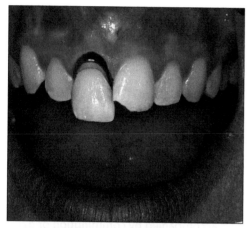

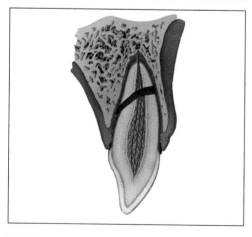

When did the injury occur?

The answer will reveal a time factor, which is critical when considering treatment of avulsed or displaced teeth as the time factor can have a direct influence on the choice of treatment.

Where did the injury occur?

While there might be legal implications in this answer, this will also indicate the possibility of contamination of wounds.

How did the injury occur?

The answer to this question will indicate possible zones of injury (e.g. crown-root fractures in the premolar and molar region after impact to the chin). Any inconsistency between the wounds observed in a child and the history provided should raise suspicion of child abuse and call for the assistance of other medical specialties. Also a marked treatment delay should raise the suspicion of child abuse.

Was there a period of unconsciousness?

If so, how long? Is there headache? Amnesia? Nausea? Vomiting? These are all signs of brain concussion and require medical attention and sometimes observation at a hospital. However, this usually does not contraindicate emergency treatment of the dental injury (e.g. replantation of avulsed teeth).

Have there been previous injuries to the teeth?

Answers to this may explain radiographic findings, such as pulp canal obliteration and incomplete root formation in a dentition with otherwise completed root development.

What measures have been taken at the place of accident or another clinic?

Teeth may have been replanted or stored in media after the accident. The patient may also have been referred from another emergency clinic and it is of importance to document what has been done at the other clinic.

Is there a change in occlusion?

An affirmative answer could imply tooth luxation, alveolar fracture, jaw fracture, or luxation or fracture of the temporomandibular joint.

Is there an increased reaction in the teeth to cold and/or heat?

A positive finding indicates exposure of dentin and need of dentinal coverage.

Medical history

Finally, a short medical history should reveal possible allergies, blood disorders, medication and other information that may influence treatment. Ask also if the patient is covered by antitetanus vaccination.

Traumatic Dental Injuries: A Manual, Third Edition   © J.O. Andreasen, L.K. Bakland, M.T. Flores, F.M. Andreasen and L. Andersson
Published 2011 by Blackwell Publishing Ltd

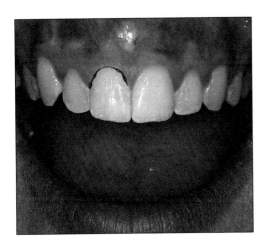

CLINICAL EXAMINATION

Examine from outside and progress inward, i.e. start with inspecting and palpating extraoral soft tissue and underlying bone. The penetrating nature of wounds and presence of foreign bodies should be determined. Intraoral soft tissue and bone is inspected and palpated. Appendices 1 and 2 show standardized clinical examination forms that will aid the clinician in an orderly examination. Thereafter, the hard dental tissues are examined for the presence of *infractions* and *fractures*. Directing the examination light beam parallel to the labial surface of the injured tooth facilitates the diagnosis of *infractions*. In cases of crown fractures, pulp exposures should be detected and their size noted. Moreover, concomitant luxation injuries (i.e. in connection with crown and root fractures) should be recorded, as these have a negative influence on long-term prognosis with respect to pulpal healing.

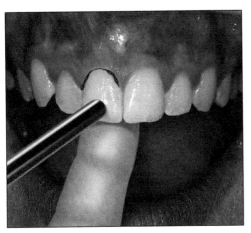

MOBILITY TEST

Mobility testing should determine the extent of loosening, especially axially, of individual teeth (an indication of disrupted pulpal vascularity) and mobility of groups of teeth (an indication of alveolar fracture). The *degree of mobility* is registered on a scale of 0–3 (0 = no loosening, 1 = horizontal loosening ≤1 mm, 2 = horizontal loosening ≥1 mm, 3 = axial loosening) and is an aid in defining the type of luxation.[21] It is important, however, to distinguish between normal physiologic mobility and no mobility which is found in cases of intrusion and lateral luxation at the time of injury, or ankylosis in the follow-up period. '0' mobility should, therefore, be used in conjunction with *percussion testing* in order to distinguish between normal physiologic mobility and no mobility (see below).

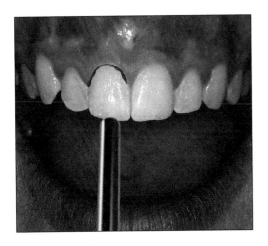

PERCUSSION TEST

Percussion testing, with a finger in small children or the handle of a metal instrument, has two functions. *Tenderness to percussion* will indicate damage to the PDL. Percussion of the labial surface will yield either a high or low *percussion tone*. A high, metallic tone implies that the injured tooth is locked into bone (as in lateral luxation or intrusion). At the follow-up examinations, this tone indicates ankylosis. This finding can be confirmed if a finger is placed on the lingual surface of the tooth to be tested. It is possible to feel the tapping of the instrument on a tooth with a normal PDL. In cases of intrusion, lateral luxation or ankylosis, percussion is not easily felt through the tooth tested.

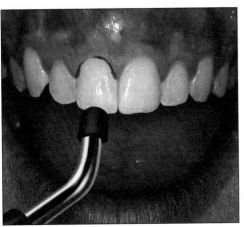

PULPAL SENSIBILITY TESTING

Electrometric sensibility testing should be carried out whenever possible as it yields important information about the neurovascular supply to the pulp of involved teeth.[20,21] The most reliable response is obtained when the electrode is placed on the incisal edge or the most incisal aspect of enamel (with crown fractures). It should be noted that young teeth with incomplete root formation do not respond consistently to sensibility testing or at higher threshold values compared with teeth with completed root formation. However, the response at the time of injury provides a baseline value for comparison at later follow-up examinations. Finally, sensibility testing in the primary dentition may yield inconclusive information due to a lack of patient cooperation.

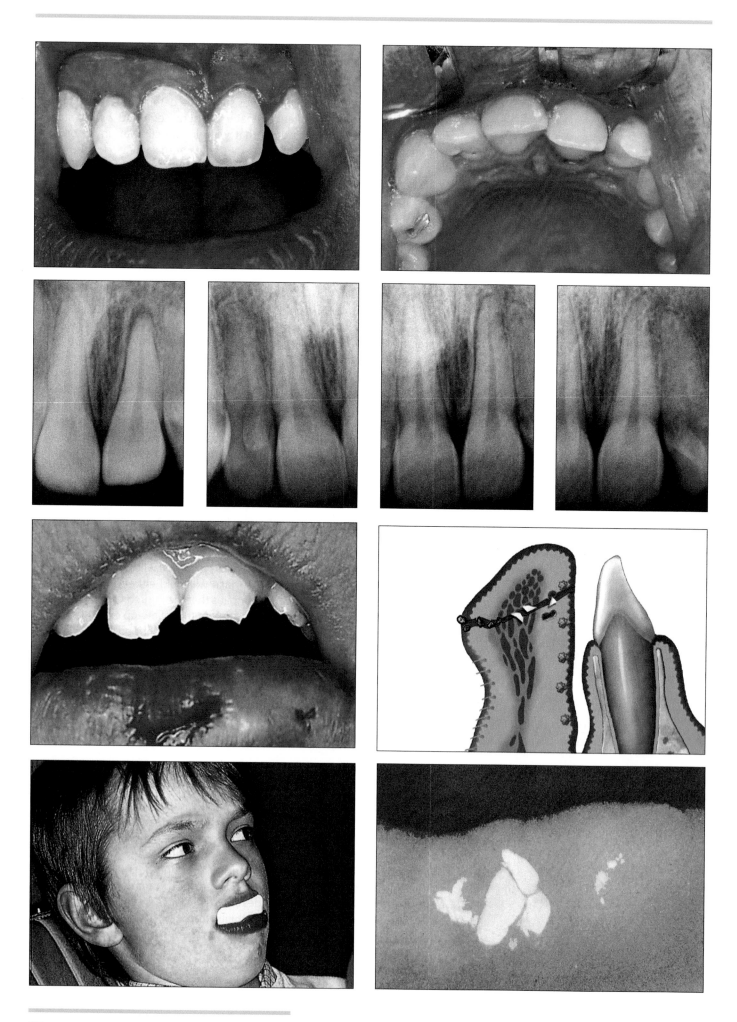

RADIOGRAPHIC EXAMINATION

The clinical examination, which has focused on the area of injury, is followed by a radiographic examination.

Several studies have demonstrated the importance of multiple radiographic exposures for revealing tooth displacement at the time of injury as well as periapical pathosis at the follow-up visits.[21] Radiographic film format is worth considering in order to achieve high quality, reproducible images. A steep occlusal exposure (using a size 2 film [DF 58, EP 21] or a similar sized sensor for digital radiography) of the traumatized anterior region gives an excellent view of most *lateral luxations, apical and mid-root fractures and alveolar fractures*. The standard periapical bisecting angle exposure of each traumatized tooth (using a size 1 film [DF 56, EP 11] or sensor provides information about *cervical root fractures* as well as other tooth displacements. Thus, a radiographic examination comprising one steep occlusal exposure and three periapical bisecting angle exposures of the traumatized region will provide sufficient information in determining the extent of trauma. It should also be pointed out that cone beam CT will provide exceedingly revealing information about all types of dental injuries and if available this technology should be recommended.[20,23]

Panoramic radiographs (OPG) give excellent overviews and reveal mandibular fractures. When mid-face fractures are suspected CT scans may be required which are usually carried out at a hospital.

RADIOGRAPHIC EXAMINATION OF SOFT TISSUE INJURIES

In the presence of a *penetrating lip wound*, a soft tissue radiograph is indicated in order to locate any foreign bodies.[20] It should be noted that the orbicularis oris muscles close tightly around foreign bodies in the lip, making them impossible to palpate; they can only be identified radiographically. This is accomplished by placing a dental film between the lips and the dental arch and using 25% of the normal exposure time. If this exposure reveals foreign bodies (a radiographic examination will normally demonstrate foreign bodies such as tooth fragments, composite filling material, metal and gravel, whereas organic materials such as cloth and wood cannot be seen), a lateral radiograph can be added (at 50% normal exposure time) to visualize the foreign bodies in relation to the cutaneous and mucosal surfaces of the lips. With the combined information from the clinical and radiographic examinations, diagnosis, prognosis and treatment planning can then be accomplished.

Finally, *photographic registration* of the trauma is recommended, as it offers an exact documentation of the extent of injury and can be used later in treatment planning, legal claims or clinical research.

FOLLOW-UP

A well-designed follow-up procedure is essential to diagnose complications. The following recall schedule has been found suitable in this regard:

- *1–2 weeks*. Only for patients with replanted teeth. Splint removal should in most cases be performed after 2 weeks. In cases where the PDL has been removed, 4 weeks splinting is recommended.
- *3–4 weeks*. A radiographic examination may demonstrate periapical radiolucencies and in some instances inflammatory resorption.
- *6–8 weeks*. A radiographic and clinical examination is able to demonstrate most cases of pulp necrosis as well as inflammatory root resorption.
- *2 and 6 months*. Optional for cases with questionable healing.
- *1 year*. A clinical and radiographic examination can provide information for the long-term prognosis. Special trauma entities such as root fractures, intrusions and replanted teeth may require longer observation periods.

NOTES

Diagnosis of Pulpal Healing Complications

┌─ OBJECTIVES ───┐

1   Recognize the clinical and radiographic signs of pulp healing, pulp necrosis and pulp canal obliteration.

2   Identify time periods following traumatic injuries when healing events can be identified.

3   Recognize the existence of transient apical breakdown.

└──┘

PULP HEALING

After a luxation injury, there may be partial or total disruption of the neurovascular supply to the pulp apically. In cases of partial disruption, reduced circulation can still be maintained throughout the pulp, with complete reconstitution of the neurovasculature after a few weeks. In cases of total rupture of the neurovascular supply, gradual revascularization will take place in an apico-coronal direction at a rate of approximately 0.5 mm vessel ingrowth per day.[6] Signs of successful revascularization are a narrowing of the pulp canal and positive sensibility testing which usually takes place after 2–3 months (Figures A–D).

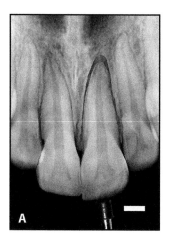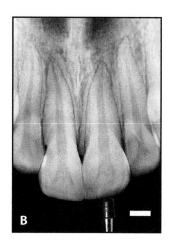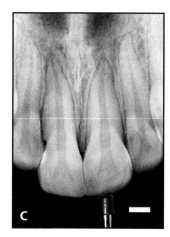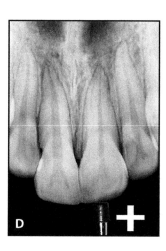

PULP NECROSIS

In cases where the injury has resulted in a partial or total rupture of the neurovascular supply to the pulp, revascularization and re-innervation processes will be initiated. Whether these processes succeed depends primarily on two factors: (1) the size of the apical foramen and (2) the presence or absence of bacteria in the healing site.[6] Unsuccessful pulpal healing with an infected pulp is evident radiographically as a periapical radiolucency, usually after 2–4 weeks (Figures A–D). In rare cases, the initial coagulation necrosis remains sterile; in these cases there will be no radiolucency. The classical signs of pulp necrosis (PN) are discoloration of the crown (gray, blue or red), negative sensibility testing and apical radiolucency, as well as persistent tenderness to percussion. Moreover, with immature teeth, PN can be seen as arrested root development, with or without apical closure. If two or more signs of PN are present, endodontic intervention is recommended.

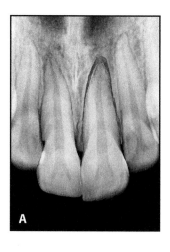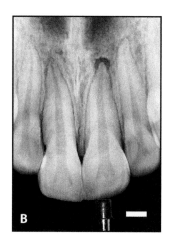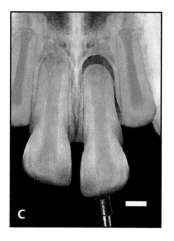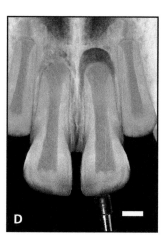

Traumatic Dental Injuries: A Manual, Third Edition   © J.O. Andreasen, L.K. Bakland, M.T. Flores, F.M. Andreasen and L. Andersson
Published 2011 by Blackwell Publishing Ltd

PULP CANAL OBLITERATION

In cases where the injury causes severance of the neurovascular supply to the pulp, healing implies revascularization and re-innervation of the ischemic pulp (see page 11). If this process succeeds, hard tissue deposition along the pulp canal walls resumes, however, at an accelerated pace.[24] This type of pulp response is frequent in all types of luxation injuries involving displacement especially in young permanent teeth with incomplete root formation. Within 1 year, an almost totally obliterated pulp canal may be seen (Figures A–C). Such a tooth runs a 1% annual risk of developing pulp necrosis (Figure D).[25,26] The cause for this event has not yet been determined.

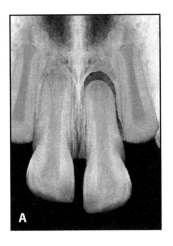
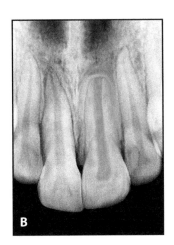
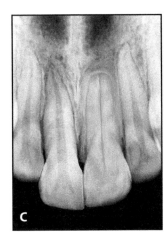
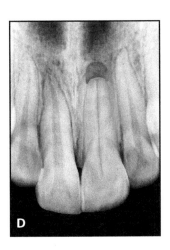

TRANSIENT APICAL BREAKDOWN

When the injury has resulted in severance of the neurovascular supply to the pulp and the apical foramen is narrow, the revascularization process will also engage osteoclastic activity in the base of the socket and the apical foramen in order to create space for ingrowth of new tissue (Figures A–C).[27] This process is transient; and when revascularization is complete, the radiolucent area will disappear (Figure D). This process is usually seen 2–12 months after injury and usually involves extruded and laterally luxated young permanent teeth.

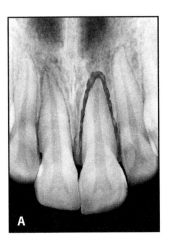
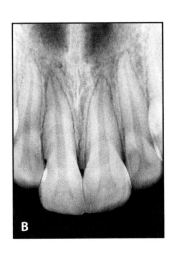
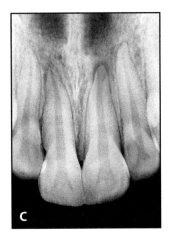
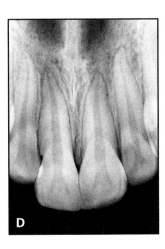

Diagnosis of Periodontal Healing Complications

OBJECTIVES

1   Recognize the radiographic signs of the three resorption types which may affect the root surface after trauma.

2   Identify time periods following traumatic injuries when the various resorption types are likely to occur.

3   Recognize the existence of transient marginal breakdown.

REPAIR-RELATED RESORPTION (SURFACE RESORPTION)

This resorption entity represents the healing response to a localized injury in the PDL, affecting the cells adjacent to the root surface (see page 12). The typical situation where repair-related resorption occurs appears to be concussion and lateral luxation (Figures A–D).[28,29] It can also occur following intru-sion and replantation, where it may affect all parts of the root, and in root fractures, where it is seen next to the fracture line.[30] Repair-related resorption is typically identified 4 weeks after injury.

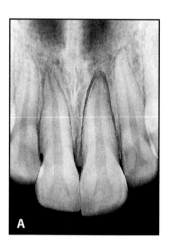
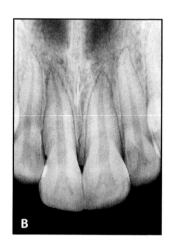
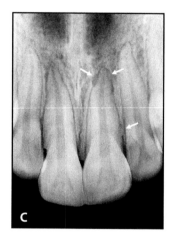
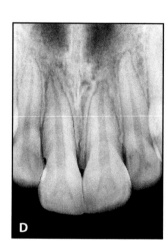

INFECTION-RELATED RESORPTION (INFLAMMATORY RESORPTION)

This resorption entity represents a combined injury to the pulp and the PDL, and where bacteria primarily located in the root canal and dentinal tubules trigger osteoclastic activity on the root surface (see page 12). This type of resorption can affect all parts of the root and is especially common after intrusion and replantation of avulsed teeth. Infection-related resorption is typically diagnosed 2–4 weeks after injury.[28,29] This type of resorption is a rapidly progressing process that may result in total resorption of the root within a month in young, immature teeth (Figure A–D).

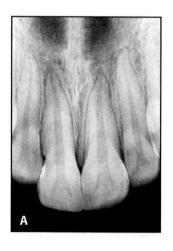
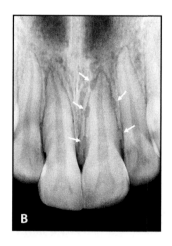
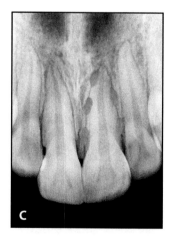
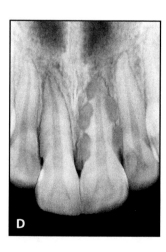

Traumatic Dental Injuries: A Manual, Third Edition   © J.O. Andreasen, L.K. Bakland, M.T. Flores, F.M. Andreasen and L. Andersson
Published 2011 by Blackwell Publishing Ltd

ANKYLOSIS-RELATED RESORPTION (REPLACEMENT RESORPTION)

This resorption process is in response to extensive damage to the innermost layer of the PDL. Due to the predominant healing response from the socket wall, an ankylosis is formed (see page 13). Due to skeletal remodeling, the root structure is gradually replaced by bone at a rate comparable to the general bone remodeling speed in the patient (Figures B–D).[28,29] Ankylosis occurs frequently after intrusions and after replantation of avulsed teeth. It can usually be diagnosed radiographically 2 months after injury; but clinically after 1 month (i.e. high percussion sound).

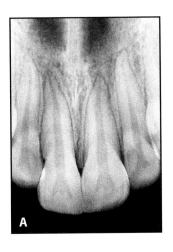
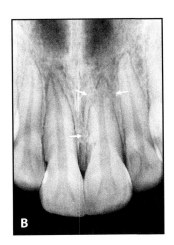
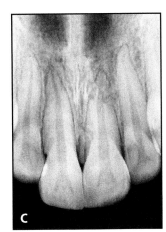
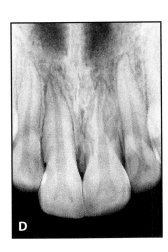

TRANSIENT MARGINAL BREAKDOWN

Where there has been extensive damage to the bony part of the socket, resorption of the injured socket wall must take place prior to healing. This event may occur after lateral luxation and intrusion, and can be seen radiographically as resorption of the lamina dura and clinically as granulation tissue in the gingival area. After 1 month, this process will resolve with later reformation of socket bone (Figures A–D).

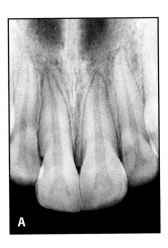
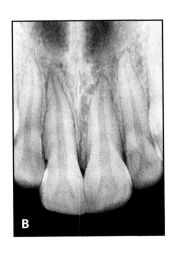
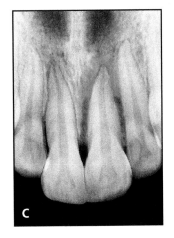
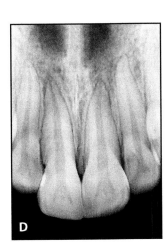

Treatment Priorities after Dental Trauma

OBJECTIVE

1 To define trauma conditions that should be treated acutely (i.e. within a few hours), or can be treated subacutely (i.e. within 24 hours) or delayed (i.e. after 24 hours).

TREATMENT PRIORITIES

It has been commonly assumed that all injuries should be treated on an emergency basis. This was for the comfort of the patient and to reduce wound healing complications. For reasons of practicality and for the best use of resources, priorities can be assigned to various types of injuries. *Acute treatment priority* would be given to those injuries that would benefit from treatment within a few hours; *subacute treatment priority* would be given to those injuries in which treatment delays of up to *24 hours* are not likely to affect healing outcomes; and *delayed treatment priority* would be for injuries for which treatment delayed more than 24 hours would be acceptable. Intra-oral treatment is difficult if the lips are sutured first. For this reason, suturing of lip lesions should be performed after intra-oral treatment has been completed. The following classification into these three categories is based on a recent study of the effect of treatment delay on the various trauma entities.[31]

ACUTE TREATMENT PRIORITY

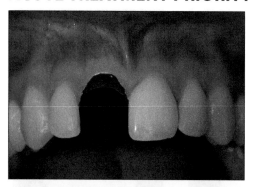

TOOTH AVULSION

A very strong relationship has been found between healing outcome and storage condition and storage time (see page 53). Tooth avulsion should therefore be considered an acute trauma situation, at least if the tooth has not already been replanted.

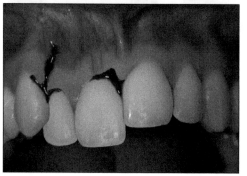

ALVEOLAR FRACTURE

In one clinical study a significant relationship was found between the occurrence of pulp necrosis and treatment delay of more than 3 hours.[32] Immediate repositioning and splinting is recommended to alleviate pain and discomfort due to occlusal interference.

EXTRUSION, LATERAL LUXATION AND ROOT FRACTURE

At present there are only a few studies that have examined the effect of treatment delay on pulpal healing after luxation injuries and root fractures. One study of luxated teeth has shown a significant difference in healing after a treatment delay of 5 hours. Other studies have shown a difference between treatment delays for 33 hours and more.[31] A recent study of 400 root fractures could not verify an effect of early treatment.[33] Until new research shows otherwise, these traumas should be considered candidates for acute treatment to alleviate the patient's pain due to occlusal interference.

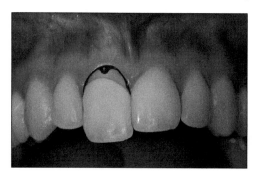
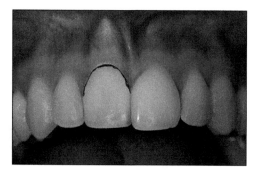
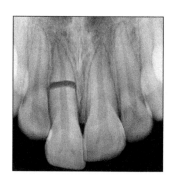

Traumatic Dental Injuries: A Manual, Third Edition   © J.O. Andreasen, L.K. Bakland, M.T. Flores, F.M. Andreasen and L. Andersson
Published 2011 by Blackwell Publishing Ltd

SUBACUTE TREATMENT PRIORITY

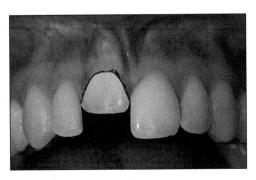

INTRUSION

A clinical study has shown almost identical healing results of immediate (surgical) repositioning and delayed orthodontic repositioning.[31] It therefore seems reasonable to use a subacute approach for this trauma entity.

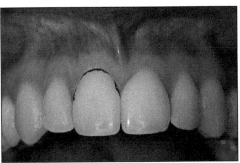

CONCUSSION, SUBLUXATION

A clinical study could not demonstrate a relationship between immediate treatment and pulp complications.[31] A subacute treatment approach is therefore acceptable.

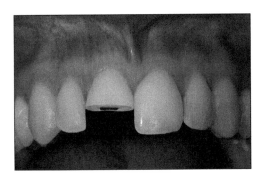

CROWN FRACTURE WITH PULP EXPOSURE

Recent clinical studies have shown that crown fractures with pulp exposure have the same long-term prognosis whether treated on an acute, subacute or delayed basis.[31] Due to the discomfort of an exposed pulp, a subacute treatment approach is therefore indicated.

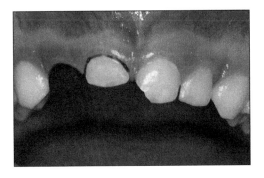

PRIMARY TEETH

Primary teeth can probably be treated with a subacute or delayed strategy unless occlusal interference due to tooth displacement indicates an acute approach to relieve symptoms.

DELAYED TREATMENT PRIORITY

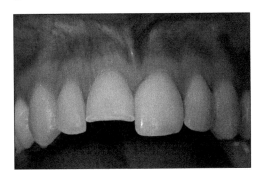

CROWN FRACTURE WITHOUT PULP EXPOSURE

Recent clinical studies have shown that crown fractures without pulp exposure have the same long-term prognosis whether treated on an acute, subacute or delayed basis.[31]

Crown Fracture without Pulp Exposure

OBJECTIVES

1 Based on clinical findings, differentiate between the types of uncomplicated crown fractures: infractions, enamel, enamel–dentin without pulp exposure.

2 Make treatment decisions based on such factors as the extent of injury, development of the tooth and status of the pulp.

3 Provide appropriate treatment for the various types of crown fractures.

4 Recognize crown fracture situations that permit fragment reattachment.

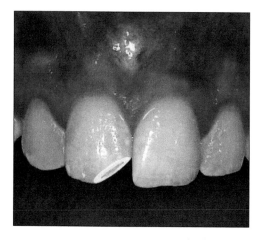

DESCRIPTION AND CLINICAL APPEARANCE

Infraction is a disruption of enamel prisms without loss of tooth substance extending from the enamel surface to the dentino–enamel junction (right lateral incisor). **Enamel fracture** is the loss of tooth substance confined to enamel (right central incisor). **Enamel–dentin fracture** (uncomplicated crown fracture) is the loss of tooth substance confined to enamel and dentin, but not involving the pulp (left central incisor).

Fractures may appear as craze lines within the enamel (infractions) or as loss of tooth substance involving only enamel or enamel and dentin. Infraction lines are usually best seen when the light beam is directed parallel to the long axis of the tooth. Besides describing only the most obvious injury (i.e. crown fracture), it is very important to diagnose concomitant luxation injuries, as these have a very significant influence on pulpal outcome.

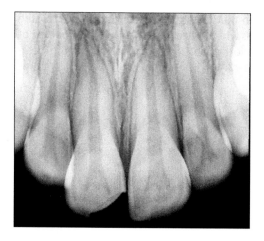

RADIOGRAPHIC APPEARANCE

The lost part of the crown can usually be recognized, whereas infraction lines cannot be seen.

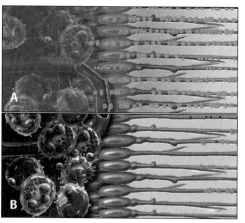

BIOLOGICAL CONSIDERATIONS AND TREATMENT PRINCIPLES

Exposed dentinal tubules can permit ingrowth of bacteria or diffusion of bacterial toxins into the pulp resulting in pulpal inflammation.[34] The severity of this response is related to pulpal vascularity, i.e. whether or not the neurovascular supply has been compromised by a concomitant luxation injury (see page 11). Arrested or compromised circulation represents an optimal situation for bacterial penetration through the dentinal tubules to the pulp (A versus B). Treatment consists primarily of protecting the pulp from external insults and restoring normal function and esthetics. If there is no associated periodontal injury (luxation), the tooth can be restored immediately using resin composites and dental adhesives. In cases of concomitant luxation injury associated with tooth mobility and gingival bleeding, a temporary restoration is indicated and a dry operative field is difficult to maintain. In these cases, care must be taken that the temporary material is not forced into the ruptured periodontal ligament space. A good sealing material appears to be glass ionomer cement.

Traumatic Dental Injuries: A Manual, Third Edition   © J.O. Andreasen, L.K. Bakland, M.T. Flores, F.M. Andreasen and L. Andersson
Published 2011 by Blackwell Publishing Ltd

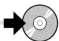

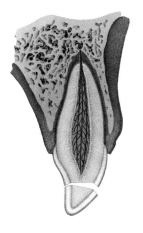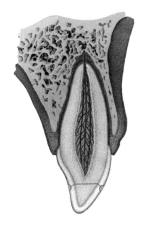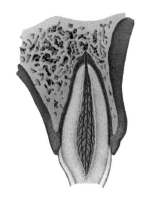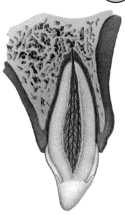

TREATMENT AND POSTOPERATIVE CONTROL

In cases of superficial enamel fractures, selective grinding of the injured tooth may be the only treatment necessary or a composite restoration can be placed.

If a crown fragment is retrieved and is without significant substance loss, it can be reattached using dental adhesives and resin composites.[34] Whether resin composite build-up or fragment reattachment is the treatment of choice, a dental adhesive should be employed. Recent laboratory studies have demonstrated that bonding strength equal to that of intact teeth can be achieved with the new bonding systems.[34]

After fragment reattachment, optimal esthetics are achieved if the fracture line facially is prepared with a double chamfer and restored with resin composite.

When using resin composite build-up, optimal esthetics and function can be achieved when the fracture edges are prepared with a 1–2 mm wide chamfer margin prior to build-up. In cases where neither of these treatments can be performed, an emergency procedure which comprises application of a temporary restoration consisting of glass ionomer cement is indicated to prevent bacterial invasion in dentin tubules.

PULP healing

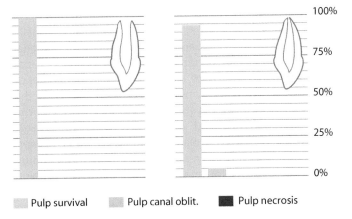

Pulp survival   Pulp canal oblit.   Pulp necrosis

PDL healing

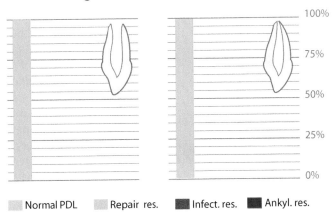

Normal PDL   Repair res.   Infect. res.   Ankyl. res.

EXPECTED OUTCOME: PULP

The tooth should be monitored 2 months and 1 year after injury. If sensibility is normal, no further control is indicated. In cases of concomitant luxation injuries, controls follow those recommended for the respective injury category.

The risk of pulpal complications is minimal. However, the risk of pulp necrosis is significantly enhanced in the case of an additional luxation injury.[35–43] Thus, it appears that the luxation diagnosis alone determines the risk of pulp necrosis.

The graphs show pulp outcome for crown fractures without luxation injuries.

EXPECTED OUTCOME: PDL

Periodontal complications are extremely rare after crown fractures and consist only of repair related resorption.[35–43]

Crown Fracture with Pulp Exposure

OBJECTIVES

1   Recognize tissue changes resulting from pulp exposure and concomitant luxation injuries.
2   Determine treatment options.
3   Provide emergency and definitive care.

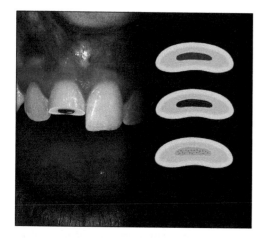

DESCRIPTION AND CLINICAL APPEARANCE

A fracture involving enamel and dentin with loss of tooth structure and exposure of the pulp (complicated crown fracture). Depending on the absence or presence of a concomitant luxation injury, the pulp will present with a bright red, cyanotic or ischemic appearance, respectively. There may be spontaneous bleeding from the pulp.

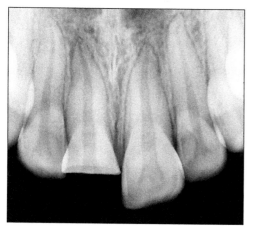

RADIOGRAPHIC APPEARANCE

Lost tooth substance is apparent, as well as periodontal changes in the case of concomitant luxation.

BIOLOGICAL CONSIDERATIONS

Exposed pulp tissue has a very good healing capacity in that it can normally close the perforation by forming a dentin barrier if a proper capping material is used.[39,44–48] Clinical studies have shown that the length of exposure (days or weeks) does not reduce the chance of hard tissue healing.[47,48] Immediate or delayed treatment in the form of pulp capping or partial pulpotomy is the best solution when possible. This implies that the pulp can be left in the interim period before definitive treatment without a temporary coverage. Temporary coverage very often shows microleakage with penetration of anerobic bacteria into the exposed pulp, which represent a very harmful condition which may lead to an infected partial or total pulp necrosis. Proper capping or amputation materials appear to be calcium hydroxide compounds and mineral trioxide aggregate (MTA), both of which have been found to lead to a hard tissue bridging in more than 90% of cases.[44–48,188] When pulp capping or partial pulpotomy is performed (Figure A) with calcium hydroxide as the amputation material (shaded area), the following healing events will occur.[47,48] Coagulation necrosis is seen in the tissue immediately beneath the calcium hydroxide (Figure B). Immediately below this zone, a wound healing response will be seen whereby new odontoblasts are differentiated and begin to form new dentin (Figure C). After 2–3 months this bridge can be detected clinically and radiographically. At this time, up to 5 μm of new dentin can be deposited daily, which means that after another 2–3 months, a significant hard tissue barrier has been formed under the pulpal wound. MTA is an alternative to calcium hydroxide and if used the coagulation zone will become very minimal and the dentin bridge will be more solid (see page 65).

Traumatic Dental Injuries: A Manual, Third Edition   © J.O. Andreasen, L.K. Bakland, M.T. Flores, F.M. Andreasen and L. Andersson
Published 2011 by Blackwell Publishing Ltd

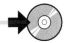

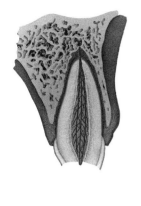

A

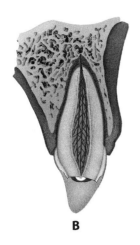

B

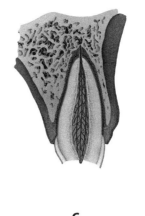

C

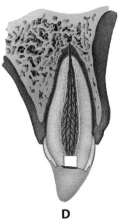

D

TREATMENT

A hard tissue barrier can be expected to be formed under the following conditions: normal pulp status prior to trauma; intact vascular supply to the pulp after trauma; the use of an appropriate pulp capping or amputation technique; and exclusion of bacteria in the pulp capping or pulp amputation zone during the healing period. If the prognosis for pulp capping is not favorable, or the absence of the pulp is preferable (i.e. due to later crown restoration and/or the placement of a post), root canal treatment is indicated. But in the case of still developing teeth, every effort should be made to preserve the pulp for continued root development.

PULP CAPPING

The tooth is isolated with rubber dam and the fracture surface is cleaned with chlorhexidine and sodium hypochlorite. Calcium hydroxide paste is applied only to the pulpal wound (A, B). Thereafter, the tooth can be restored either with dentin adhesive and conventional resin composite build-up or fragment reattachment. In the latter case space should be made in the coronal fragment for the pulp capping paste.[48]

Radiographic evidence of hard tissue healing can be seen 3 months after treatment.

PARTIAL PULPOTOMY

The tooth is anesthetized, isolated with rubber dam and the fracture surface cleaned with chlorhexidine. Preferably using a round carbide bur or diamond mounted in an air rotor with copious water spray, the pulp is removed to a depth of 2–3 mm, creating a box-like cavity (C,D). Once complete hemostasis is achieved, a thin layer of calcium hydroxide paste or MTA (see page 64) is applied to the wound and compressed slightly. Over this, and still within the prepared cavity, a thin layer of resin-modified glass ionomer cement is applied. Thereafter, the tooth can be restored using dental adhesive with either conventional resin composite build-up or crown fragment reattachment.[48] Radiographic examination should be made to detect signs of pulp necrosis or pulp canal obliteration (both rare findings in cases of fracture without concomitant luxation injury).

PULP healing

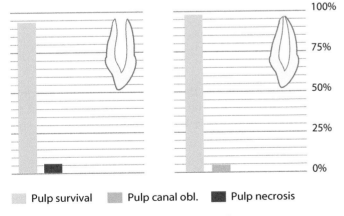

Pulp survival   Pulp canal obl.   Pulp necrosis

PDL healing

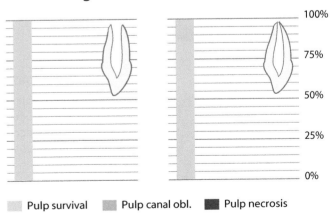

Pulp survival   Pulp canal obl.   Pulp necrosis

EXPECTED OUTCOME: PULP CAPPING

Long-term studies have shown very high success rates of pulp capping and partial pulpotomy with respect to pulp survival.[41–48] Radiographic evidence of hard tissue closure of the perforation can be seen 3 months after treatment. The tooth should be followed 1 and 5 years after injury and monitored for pulpal sensibility. When using resin composite build-up, the pulp tester should be placed on the most incisal

aspect of the available enamel. The graphs show pulp outcome for crown fractures without luxation injuries.

EXPECTED OUTCOME: PARTIAL PULPOTOMY

Long-term studies have shown very high success rates for partial pulpotomy with respect to pulp survival irrespective of the stage of root development.[47]

Crown-Root Fracture

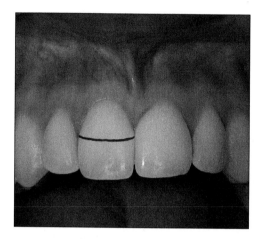

DESCRIPTION AND CLINICAL APPEARANCE

This is a fracture involving enamel, dentin and cementum, with or without pulpal involvement.

The fracture usually starts at the mid-portion of the crown facially and extends below the gingival level palatally. The coronal fragment is more or less displaced in an incisal direction, which results in pain from occlusion. In the premolar and molar regions, the fracture is usually confined to the buccal or palatal cusps.

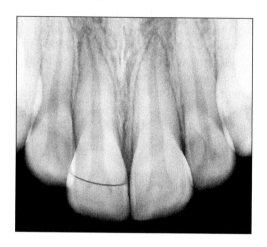

RADIOGRAPHIC APPEARANCE

With labio-lingual fractures only the incisal and labial part of the fracture can be identified, whereas the lingual and more apically placed part of the fracture usually cannot be seen due to the hinge-like displacement of the fragment. Typically, proximal crown-root fractures are evident radiographically.

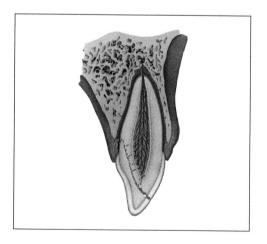

BIOLOGICAL CONSIDERATIONS

The histological events in the pulp mimic those of complicated and uncomplicated crown fractures, depending on the location of the fracture. Due to plaque accumulation in the line of fracture, the PDL next to the fracture line also shows inflammatory changes.[49]

Traumatic Dental Injuries: A Manual, Third Edition　© J.O. Andreasen, L.K. Bakland, M.T. Flores, F.M. Andreasen and L. Andersson
Published 2011 by Blackwell Publishing Ltd

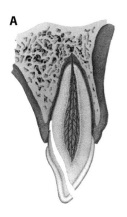
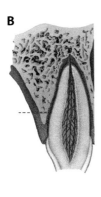
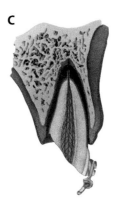
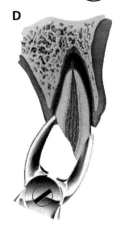

A   B   C   D

TREATMENT PRINCIPLES

Under ideal conditions treatment principles include sealing of exposed dentinal tubules, protecting the pulp, and restoring the tooth to its original function and esthetics.[49,50]

The extent of the fracture below the gingival margin, as related to the length and morphology of the root, dictates the treatment chosen. The primary goal is to create a situation where the tooth can be restored after removal of the coronal fragment. In some cases, the apical fragment can be left in position and the tooth restored with or without exposing the subgingival aspect of the fracture; or the tooth can be surgically or orthodontically extruded into a position where restoration is possible. All forms of treatment can be performed either immediately or after some days' or weeks' delay. If treatment must be postponed, the coronal fragment can be temporarily splinted to adjacent teeth using an acid etch technique and composite resin. Immobilization of the loose fragment will alleviate symptoms and permit the patient to be comfortable until the definitive treatment can be performed.

FRAGMENT REMOVAL AND GINGIVAL REATTACHMENT (FIGURE A)

The coronal fragment is removed and the gingiva is allowed to reattach to the exposed dentin (i.e. by formation of a long junctional epithelium). After some weeks, the tooth can be restored above gingival level.

FRAGMENT REMOVAL AND SURGICAL EXPOSURE OF SUBGINGIVAL FRACTURE (FIGURE B)

If the fracture extends below the alveolar crest, the subgingival fracture is exposed by gingivectomy and/or osteotomy after removal of the coronal fragment. Following gingival healing, the tooth is restored with a post-retained crown. While this procedure might appear to be most rational, long-term esthetic success can be compromised due to an accumulation of granulation tissue in the gingival sulcus palatally, which can lead to labial migration of the restored tooth.[51]

FRAGMENT REMOVAL AND ORTHODONTIC EXTRUSION (FIGURE C)

The coronal fragment is initially stabilized to adjacent teeth. Pulp extirpation and canal obturation with gutta-percha and sealer can be performed at a later appointment. The coronal fragment is then removed and the tooth extruded over a 4–6 week period. The tooth should be slightly over extruded (0.5 mm), due to risk of relapse. A labial gingivectomy is then performed 1 mm apical to the expected future gingival level in order to compensate for the expected re-growth of the gingiva[49], after which the tooth can be restored.

FRAGMENT REMOVAL AND SURGICAL EXTRUSION (FIGURE D)

After removing the coronal fragment, the root is loosened with elevators and forceps and repositioned in a more incisal position, so that the entire fracture surface is exposed above the gingival level.[52–57] In some cases a 90° or 180° rotation of the root may be an advantage to ensure minimum exposure of the root surface in the oral cavity. The root fragment is then stabilized with sutures or a non-rigid splint. The pulp is extirpated and the entrance to the root canal is sealed with temporary cement. After 4 weeks, when the tooth is stabilized in its socket, endodontic treatment is completed; and after another 4–5 weeks, the tooth can be restored.

PARTIAL OR TOTAL TOOTH REMOVAL

This is indicated in cases of fractures that extend so deep below the gingival margin that the crown–root ratio after extrusion does not allow a crown restoration. In case of children with residual alveolar growth a decoronation procedure may be performed to preserve the volume of the alveolar process to original function and esthetics.[49]

Root Fracture

OBJECTIVES

1 Recognize the tissues involved.
2 Define objectives for acute treatment.
3 Describe healing outcomes based on a clinical and radiographic evaluation.
4 Describe treatment options for healing complications.

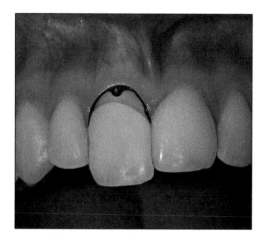

DESCRIPTION AND CLINICAL APPEARANCE

Root fracture involves dentin, cementum and the pulp. They can be further classified based on the type of displacement of the coronal fragment (see Luxation Injuries on page 17). Clinically, the tooth appears elongated and is usually displaced palatally. Transient crown discoloration (red or gray) may occur.

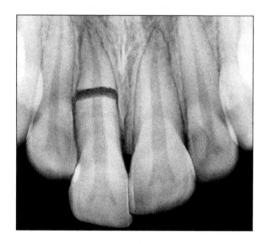

RADIOGRAPHIC APPEARANCE

Radiolucent lines separate the root into two or more fragments. The apical fragment is always left *in situ*, whereas the coronal fragment is often displaced. It should be noted that in cases where there is minimal luxation (i.e. concussion, subluxation) of the coronal fragment, the root fracture may not be evident until a later radiographic examination.

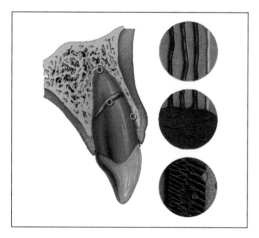

BIOLOGICAL CONSIDERATIONS AND TREATMENT PRINCIPLES

This is a complex injury to the PDL, pulp, dentin and cementum. The injury to the coronal segment can be considered a luxation injury, with resultant trauma to the PDL and neurovascular supply to the coronal pulp. In contrast, the apical fragment remains essentially uninjured.[58–60] To facilitate healing, optimal repositioning is considered essential. A splinting period of 4 weeks appears to be sufficient in most cases to secure healing.[58–60] In cases of root fracture with associated luxation, the displaced coronal fragment should be gently repositioned.[61] This procedure is usually not painful, thus rarely indicating the use of local anesthesia. After repositioning, a control radiograph is taken. The tooth is then splinted. A semi-rigid splint should be used for 4 weeks. In case of fractures located to the cervical region a longer splinting period (e.g. 4 months) may be indicated although no conclusive evidence exists.[62] It is advisable to monitor healing for at least 1 year to determine pulpal status.

Traumatic Dental Injuries: A Manual, Third Edition   © J.O. Andreasen, L.K. Bakland, M.T. Flores, F.M. Andreasen and L. Andersson
Published 2011 by Blackwell Publishing Ltd

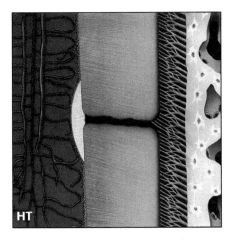
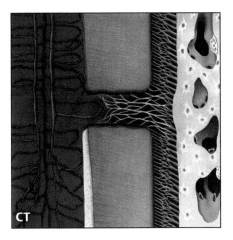
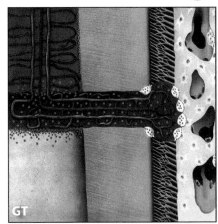

HEALING EVENTS AFTER ROOT FRACTURE

Healing outcomes after root fracture can be divided into three groups:

- *Hard tissue healing (HT),* where dentin formed from odontoblasts and cementum formed from invading periodontium bridge the fracture gap (Figure A).
- *Connective tissue healing (CT),* where PDL cells invade the entire fracture gap and enclose both fragments (Figure B).
- *Interposition of granulation tissue (GT),* occurs when the necrotic coronal pulp becomes infected by bacterial invasion at the initial rupture in the PDL. Granulation tissue is then formed between the two fragments as a response to the infected coronal root canal (Figure C).[58,63] When GT is successfully treated endodontically (coronal fragment), optimally with a calcium hydroxide interim dressing followed by gutta percha root filling or MTA, healing will take place as CT.[64,65]

The following clinical and radiographic signs can be recorded, which indicate type of healing:

- *HT:* normal tooth mobility, normal pulpal sensibility, slightly discernible fracture line and an intact coronal pulp canal can be seen radiographically.
- *CT:* increased mobility of the involved coronal fragment, normal pulpal sensibility, markedly discernible fracture line and obliteration of the coronal pulp canal radiographically.
- *GT:* increased to excessive mobility of the involved tooth, usually extrusion, negative pulpal sensibility, increasing radiographic distance between fragments and bone resorption (radiolucency) at the level of fracture.[58]

PULP healing

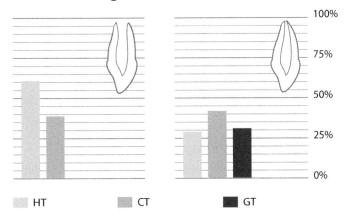

100%
75%
50%
25%
0%

| HT | CT | GT |

PDL healing

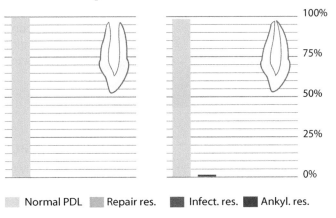

100%
75%
50%
25%
0%

| Normal PDL | Repair res. | Infect. res. | Ankyl. res. |

EXPECTED OUTCOME: PULP

The most significant factor determining healing events appears to be the stage of root development at the time of injury and the extent of initial displacement (luxation) of the coronal fragment.[59, 60, 66–68] In immature teeth, healing with HT is very frequent, whereas in mature teeth, healing by CT and non-healing with GT predominate.[59, 60, 66–68] Moreover, HT is related to fractures with an intact pulp from the time of injury (concussion, subluxation). CT is related to moderate pulpal damage due to minor displacement of the coronal fragment (extrusion, lateral luxation) and in cases of incomplete repositioning.[60]

EXPECTED OUTCOME: PDL

Resorption within the coronal pulp canal next to the fracture line can often be seen as part of the HT and CT healing process; this process should be considered remodeling and should not be confused with GT.[58] When the resorption processes are seen to extend into bone adjacent to the line of fracture, repair-related resorption in the peripheral part of the fracture is a very frequent finding.

Alveolar Process Fracture

OBJECTIVES

1 Recognize injury by appropriate clinical and radiographic examination.

2 Identify the various dental, periodontal and alveolar elements involved in the injury.

3 Define objectives of acute treatment.

4 Describe healing outcomes.

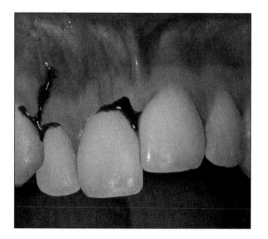

DESCRIPTION AND CLINICAL APPEARANCE

This trauma entity is a fracture of the alveolar process, which may or may not involve alveolar sockets.

The typical clinical appearance is often one in which a segment containing one or more teeth is displaced axially or laterally, usually resulting in occlusal disturbance.[69,70] When mobility testing is performed, the entire fragment is found to be mobile (several teeth move as a unit), and a percussion test gives a dull sound. Gingival lacerations are frequently observed.

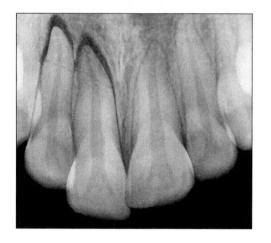

RADIOGRAPHIC APPEARANCE

A fracture line can usually be seen, depending on the angle of the central radiographic beam. The horizontal part of the fracture line may be found in all locations, ranging from the cervical to the apical or periapical region. A differential diagnosis must be made with root fracture. Change in the angulation of the central beam in a root fracture will not alter the fracture position on the root surface. In cases of alveolar fractures, however, the fracture line will move up or down along to the root surface according to the X-ray beam angulation. A panoramic exposure is of great help in determining the course and position of fracture lines. If available a cone beam CT technique is recommended to get a full set of labio-lingual information about the fracture.

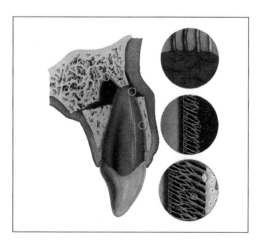

BIOLOGICAL CONSIDERATIONS AND TREATMENT PRINCIPLES

The bony fracture may disrupt vascular supply to the associated teeth which can result in pulp necrosis. Due to frequent concomitant luxation injury and damage to the PDL, root resorption can sometimes occur.[69]

The treatment principles comprise repositioning and immobilization of the displaced bone–tooth fragment and monitoring of pulp vitality.

Traumatic Dental Injuries: A Manual, Third Edition © J.O. Andreasen, L.K. Bakland, M.T. Flores, F.M. Andreasen and L. Andersson
Published 2011 by Blackwell Publishing Ltd

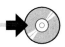

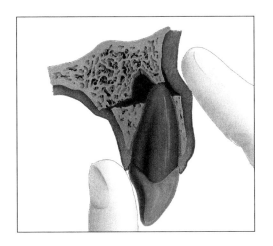

TREATMENT

Using infiltration or preferably a regional block anesthesia, the fragment is repositioned. As with lateral luxation, it is sometimes necessary to disengage the apices of the involved teeth from a bony lock. This is done via apical digital pressure or an initial axial traction of the fracture segment. The fractured segment is splinted with a semi-rigid splint (see page 62).

The splint is removed after 3–4 weeks. Pulpal and PDL healing should be monitored after 4 weeks, 8 weeks and 6 months and after 1 year and yearly for 5 years.[71,72]

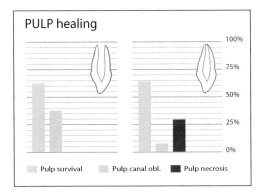

PULP healing

100%
75%
50%
25%
0%

Pulp survival　　Pulp canal obl.　■ Pulp necrosis

EXPECTED OUTCOME: PULP

Pulp necrosis is a frequent finding in teeth with associated alveolar socket fracture.[71-73]

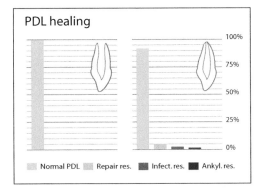

PDL healing

100%
75%
50%
25%
0%

Normal PDL　　Repair res.　■ Infect. res.　■ Ankyl. res.

EXPECTED OUTCOME: PDL

Root resorption is a rare finding.[71-73]

NOTES

Concussion

OBJECTIVES

1 Differentiate type of luxation injury.
2 Identify injured tissues involved.
3 Define objectives of initial treatment.
4 Estimate frequency and type of possible complications.

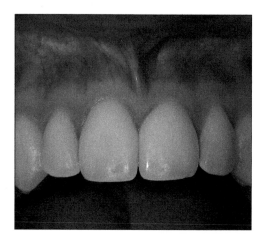

DESCRIPTION AND CLINICAL APPEARANCE

This lesion is an injury to the tooth-supporting structures without increased loosening or displacement of the tooth, but with pain to percussion.

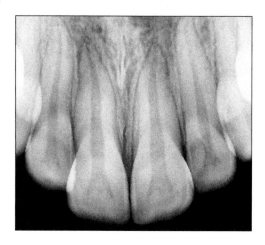

RADIOGRAPHIC APPEARANCE

The tooth is found in its normal position in the socket.

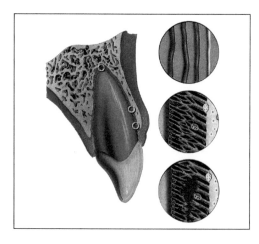

BIOLOGICAL CONSIDERATIONS

The impact results in injury to the PDL, including edema and bleeding. An added effect of the impact may be damage to the neurovascular supply to the pulp.[74]

Traumatic Dental Injuries: A Manual, Third Edition   © J.O. Andreasen, L.K. Bakland, M.T. Flores, F.M. Andreasen and L. Andersson
Published 2011 by Blackwell Publishing Ltd

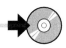

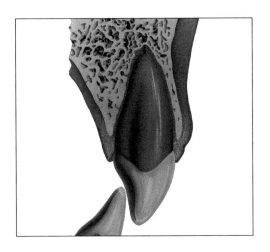

TREATMENT

No treatment is needed. However, if the tooth is in occlusion, the antagonist(s) can be slightly ground to minimize hyper-occlusion. Monitor pulpal condition for at least 1 year. Alternatively, the teeth can be splinted for patient comfort (approximately 2 weeks) or, with multiple tooth injuries, splinted according to the recommended fixation period for other injured teeth in the dental arch.[74,75]

Only a few control visits are indicated, e.g. after 4 weeks, 6–8 weeks and 1 year.

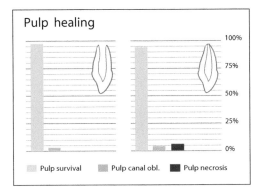

Pulp healing

- Pulp survival
- Pulp canal obl.
- Pulp necrosis

100%
75%
50%
25%
0%

EXPECTED OUTCOME: PULP

Pulpal complications are rare. Stage of root development is the decisive prognostic factor.[76, 77]

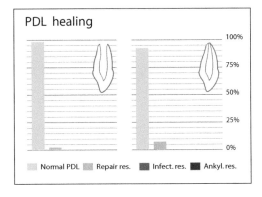

PDL healing

- Normal PDL
- Repair res.
- Infect. res.
- Ankyl. res.

100%
75%
50%
25%
0%

EXPECTED OUTCOME: PDL

Root resorption is very rare and consists exclusively in repair related resorption.[76,77]

NOTES

_____

_____

_____

_____

_____

_____

_____

_____

_____

_____

Subluxation

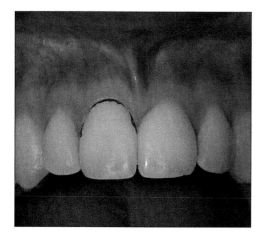

DESCRIPTION AND CLINICAL APPEARANCE

This luxation entity is an injury to the tooth-supporting structures resulting in increased mobility, but without displacement of the tooth. Bleeding from the gingival sulcus confirms the diagnosis.

A subluxated tooth (right central incisor) is mobile and there might be hemorrhage from the gingival sulcus.

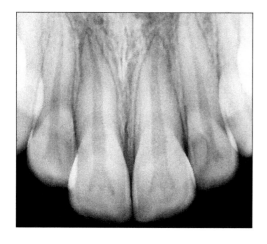

RADIOGRAPHIC APPEARANCE

The tooth is in its normal position in the socket.

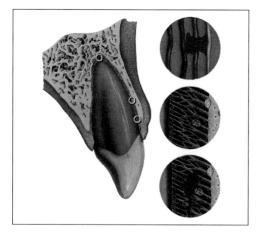

BIOLOGICAL CONSIDERATIONS

The impact results in injury to the PDL, whereby edema, bleeding and tearing of PDL fibers may occur. A secondary effect of the impact may be total or partial rupture of the neurovascular supply to the pulp.[78]

Traumatic Dental Injuries: A Manual, Third Edition   © J.O. Andreasen, L.K. Bakland, M.T. Flores, F.M. Andreasen and L. Andersson
Published 2011 by Blackwell Publishing Ltd

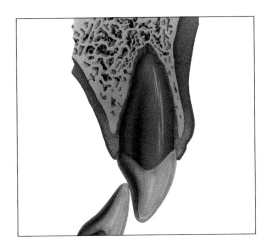

TREATMENT

If the tooth is in occlusion, the antagonist(s) can be slightly ground out of occlusion, and the patient is placed on a soft diet for 2 weeks. Alternatively, the teeth can be splinted for patient comfort (approximately 2 weeks) or, with multiple tooth injuries, splinted according to the recommended fixation period for other injured teeth in the dental arch.[78,79] Monitor pulpal response until a definitive pulpal diagnosis can be made. Only a few control visits are indicated, e.g. after 6–8 weeks and 1 year.

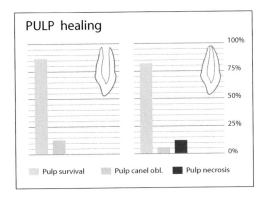

EXPECTED OUTCOME: PULP

Pulpal complications are rare. Stage of root development is the decisive prognostic factor. A significantly higher rate of pulp necrosis is found in case of an associated crown fracture.[80–82]

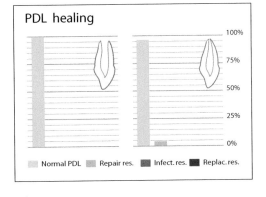

EXPECTED OUTCOME: PDL

Root resorption is very rare and when it occurs it is primarily repair-related root resorption. In very rare cases inflammatory resorption is seen.[80–82]

NOTES

Extrusive Luxation

OBJECTIVES

1 Differentiate type of luxation injury.
2 Identify injured tissues involved.
3 Define objectives of acute treatment.
4 Estimate frequency and type of complications.

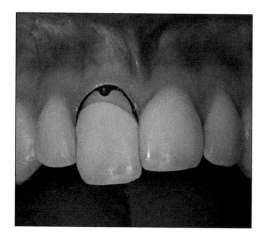

DESCRIPTION AND CLINICAL APPEARANCE

The tooth is partially displaced out of its socket.

The tooth appears elongated and is usually displaced palatally. The tooth is very loose, with bleeding from the gingival sulcus.

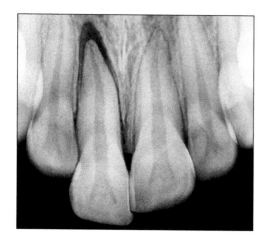

RADIOGRAPHIC APPEARANCE

The tooth appears dislocated, with the apical part of the socket empty.

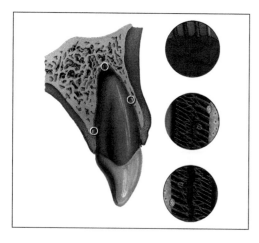

BIOLOGICAL CONSIDERATIONS AND TREATMENT PRINCIPLES

The impact results in partial disruption of the PDL attachment as well as rupture of the apical neurovascular bundle, causing increased mobility of the tooth and pulpal infarction (coagulation necrosis). The disruption of the neurovascular supply is frequently reflected in negative pulpal sensibility. Healing consists of reorganization and re-establishment of the continuity of the PDL fibers as well as pulpal revascularization and reinnervation. Pulp canal obliteration is the usual end result of successful revascularization.[83]

Optimal repositioning is the treatment goal. This will facilitate PDL healing and possibly pulpal revascularization if the apical opening is sufficiently large (at least 1 mm in diameter), as well as ensure vitality of Hertwig's epithelial root sheath and continued root development. The tooth is splinted to maintain the tooth in an anatomically correct position during the initial healing process and prevent re-extrusion.

Traumatic Dental Injuries: A Manual, Third Edition © J.O. Andreasen, L.K. Bakland, M.T. Flores, F.M. Andreasen and L. Andersson
Published 2011 by Blackwell Publishing Ltd

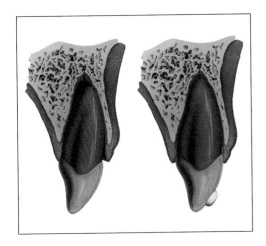

TREATMENT

The extruded tooth should be repositioned gently using axial finger pressure on the incisal edge.[84] Local anesthesia is usually not needed. When the tooth is fully repositioned, check occlusion. Stabilize the tooth for 2 weeks using a non-rigid splint (see page 62). Take a radiograph to verify correct tooth position, and monitor the pulpal condition radiographically and clinically after 2–4 weeks, 6–8 weeks, 6 months, 1 year and yearly for 5 years. If there is no sign of hard tissue changes (i.e. root resorption, bone loss), remove the splint after 2 weeks. In cases of teeth with open apices, follow-up including radiographic examination and sensibility testing for extended periods is indicated to diagnose healing complications (primarily pulp necrosis). In teeth with closed apices, the likelihood of revascularization is very reduced. Therefore, root canal therapy can be initiated just prior to splint removal. However, an exception to this practice is made for patients where continuous radiographic and pulp testing can be arranged to verify pulpal healing or necrosis, keeping in mind that if the pulp becomes infected, the root may begin to undergo infection-related resorption.[83]

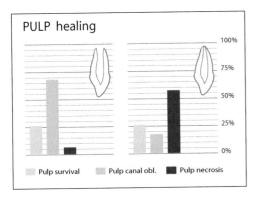

EXPECTED OUTCOME: PULP

In teeth with open apices in which revascularization takes place, pulp canal obliteration is a relatively frequent finding. Pulp necrosis is rare. In teeth with closed apices, the situation is reversed.[85–90] A significantly higher rate of pulp necrosis is found in cases that have an associated crown fracture.[88]

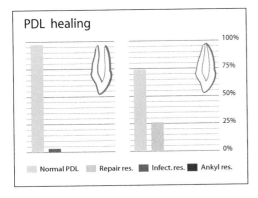

EXPECTED OUTCOME: PDL

Root resorption is rare, and then primarily repair-related resorption. However, infection-related (inflammatory) resorption can be seen, although rare, in all stages of root development in association with infected pulp necrosis.[85–90]

NOTES

43

Lateral Luxation

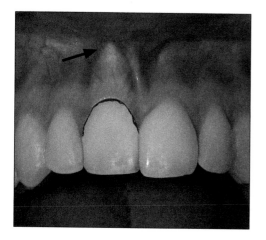

DESCRIPTION AND CLINICAL APPEARANCE

There is lateral eccentric displacement of the tooth in its socket; and it is accompanied by comminution or fracture of the alveolar bone plate (labial and/or lingual).

The crown appears displaced in its socket, usually in a palatal direction. The tooth is immobile due to its locked position in the bone, and there is a high ankylotic (metallic) percussion tone. There may or may not be bleeding from the gingival sulcus. The root apex and the displaced labial bone can be palpated in the sulcus area (arrow).

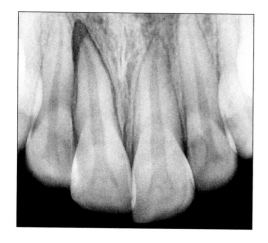

RADIOGRAPHIC APPEARANCE

A steep (occlusal) or eccentric radiographic exposure is necessary to disclose displacement. The tooth appears displaced, with the apical or lateral part of the socket empty. A periapical exposure bisecting angle may not reveal displacement.

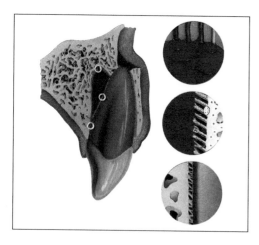

BIOLOGICAL CONSIDERATIONS AND TREATMENT PRINCIPLES

The injury is very similar to extrusive luxation. However, it is further complicated by the presence of a fracture of the labial bone plate as well as a compression zone in the cervical area palatally.[91]

Optimal repositioning is the treatment goal. This will facilitate pulpal and periodontal healing; the tooth should be splinted during the healing period due to extensive remodeling processes in the socket.

Traumatic Dental Injuries: A Manual, Third Edition   © J.O. Andreasen, L.K. Bakland, M.T. Flores, F.M. Andreasen and L. Andersson
Published 2011 by Blackwell Publishing Ltd

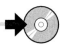

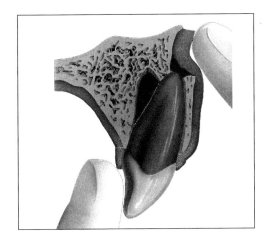

TREATMENT

The displaced tooth is usually locked firmly in its new position. Repositioning requires disengagement of the tooth from its bony lock.[91] Adequate regional anesthesia (infraorbital regional block) is necessary, as repositioning is otherwise a painful procedure. The tooth can be repositioned using forceps or digitally, with pressure in an incisal direction over the apex, whereby the tooth is first slightly extruded to disengage the apex and then repositioned in an apical direction. After repositioning, occlusion should be checked and a radiograph taken to verify correct repositioning. The tooth should be splinted for 4 weeks with a non-rigid splint. Monitor the pulpal condition and if the pulp becomes necrotic, root canal treatment is indicated to prevent root resorption. A clinical and radiographic control visit should then be performed after 2 and 4 weeks. If these controls show no sign of marginal or periradicular breakdown, the splint can be removed. If any of these signs are present, splinting should be maintained for another 4 weeks, as the tooth can be very loose at this stage of healing due to transient breakdown of the PDL. Further controls are indicated after 6–8 weeks, 6 months, 1 year and yearly for 5 years (IADT Guidelines 2007).[226]

EXPECTED OUTCOME: PULP

In teeth with open apices, observation, including radiographic examination and pulp testing, is indicated for extended periods in order to diagnose healing complications. In teeth with closed apices, the likelihood of revascularization is minimal. Therefore, root canal therapy can be initiated just prior to splint removal. However, an exception to this practice is made for patients where continuous radiographic and pulp testing can be maintained to assure healing (pulp canal obliteration and/or positive response to sensibility testing) or verify pulp necrosis (periapical lesion or symptoms of pulpitis).[91] In teeth with open apices in which revascularization occurs, pulp canal obliteration is a frequent finding, while pulp necrosis is rare. Revascularization can be confirmed radiographically by evidence of continued root formation and possibly by positive sensibility testing. In teeth with closed apices, continued lack of response to sensibility testing may indicate pulp necrosis, along with periapical rarefaction and sometimes crown discoloration.[93–99,226]

EXPECTED OUTCOME: PDL

Due to compression of the PDL, both infection-related and ankylosis-related resorption may occur; they are, however, rare. Repair-related resorption is very frequent and usually located apically.[93–99]

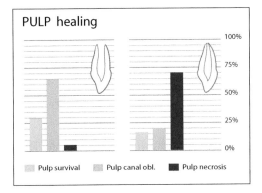

PULP healing

100%
75%
50%
25%
0%

Pulp survival   Pulp canal obl.   Pulp necrosis

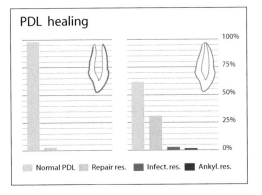

PDL healing

100%
75%
50%
25%
0%

Normal PDL   Repair res.   Infect. res.   Ankyl. res.

NOTES

_____
_____
_____
_____
_____
_____
_____
_____
_____

Intrusive Luxation

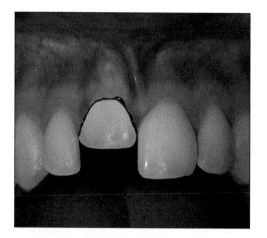

DESCRIPTION AND CLINICAL APPEARANCE

In this type of luxation the tooth is forced into the socket and locked in position in bone. This injury is accompanied by comminution or fracture of the alveolar socket.

Clinically, the crown of the tooth appears shortened. There is bleeding from the gingiva. The tooth is immobile and percussion tone is high and metallic.

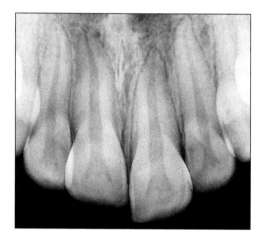

RADIOGRAPHIC APPEARANCE

The tooth appears dislocated in an apical direction with partial or complete disappearance of the periodontal ligament space. This is especially evident cervically. However, the radiographic appearance is not always diagnostic. A high ankylotic percussion tone is usually the pathognomonic feature for diagnosis.

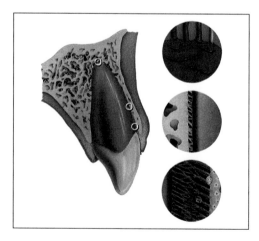

BIOLOGICAL CONSIDERATIONS AND TREATMENT PRINCIPLES

Intrusion represents a very complex wound, involving disruption of the marginal gingival seal, contusion of the alveolar bone, disruption of PDL fibers, damage to cementum, and disruption of the neurovascular supply to the pulp. Such an injury, which involves contusion (crushing) of all components of the dentoalveolar complex, implies a severely compromised healing event (see page 13). Optimal PDL healing is dependent on the presence of large non-injured areas of PDL, which is usually not the case after intrusion. Bone will, therefore, often replace the PDL and result in ankylosis (see page 10).[100,101] At present, the value of acute priority repositioning of the intruded tooth is uncertain. Spontaneous or guided re-eruption has been found to lead to healing in approximately half of the cases. However, spontaneous re-eruption can normally only be expected to occur in cases with incomplete root formation.

Traumatic Dental Injuries: A Manual, Third Edition   © J.O. Andreasen, L.K. Bakland, M.T. Flores, F.M. Andreasen and L. Andersson
Published 2011 by Blackwell Publishing Ltd

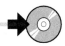

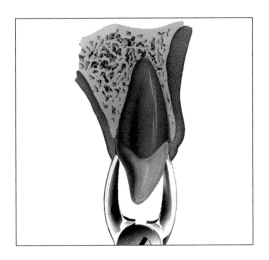

TREATMENT

Teeth with open apices. In children under the age of 16, *spontaneous repositioning* is possible and when that occurs, the outcome is the most desirable.[102–104] If no movement is noted within 3 weeks recommend rapid orthodontic repositioning. If *spontaneous repositioning* does not occur, or intrusion is more than 7 mm, one may choose to assist repositioning of the tooth surgically. Using infiltration or regional anesthesia, the tooth is grasped with forceps and slightly loosened to release it from its locked position in bone and is then left to re-erupt. Alternatively, *orthodontic extrusion* can be employed to ensure repositioning of the tooth within 3 weeks after injury, so that interceptive endodontic therapy can be initiated should pulp necrosis and/or inflammatory resorption occur. Surgical luxation can be combined with orthodontic extrusion. However, orthodontic extrusion should not be initiated the same day.

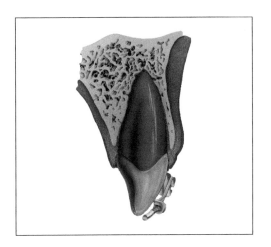

Teeth with closed apices. In these cases, spontaneous re-eruption is unreliable. The tooth should be repositioned either orthodontically or surgically as soon as possible. The pulp will likely be necrotic and root canal treatment using a short term (< 30 days) filling with calcium hydroxide is recommended. *Orthodontic extrusion* may be the treatment of choice.[102–104] If the tooth has been fully intruded, partial repositioning is necessary to permit bonding of a bracket. Extrusion should be complete within 3 weeks after injury. Prophylactic extirpation of the pulp should then be performed. A close follow-up is indicated after 2 weeks, 6–8 weeks, 6 months, 1 year and then yearly for 5 years[226], as multiple complications can occur due to the profound PDL and pulpal injuries. *Surgical repositioning* appears to be the treatment of choice for deeply intruded teeth with closed apices.[100–104] In cases of surgical repositioning, it is important that lacerated gingiva be well adapted and sutured around the cervical area of the tooth. A flexible splint should be placed and maintained for 4–8 weeks.

EXPECTED OUTCOME: PULP

Complete healing (revascularization and re-innervation) can only be expected in teeth with incomplete root formation. With increased stages of root development (closed apices), pulp necrosis is the usual outcome.[103,104] The most significant prognostic factor appears to be the stage of root development at the time of injury.[103,104]

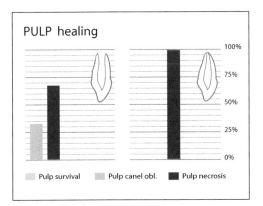

PULP healing

100%
75%
50%
25%
0%

Pulp survival   Pulp canel obl.   Pulp necrosis

EXPECTED OUTCOME: PDL

External repair, infection and ankylosis-related resorption are very frequent findings, especially in teeth with completed root development.[103–110] It should be noted that severe healing complications such as ankylosis-related root resorption can be seen as late as 5–10 years after trauma.[100]

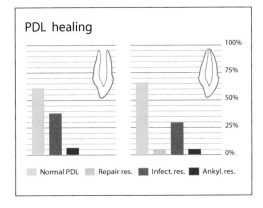

PDL healing

100%
75%
50%
25%
0%

Normal PDL   Repair res.   Infect. res.   Ankyl. res.

Avulsion

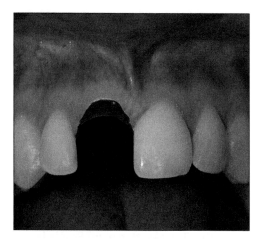

DESCRIPTION AND CLINICAL APPEARANCE

In this trauma situation, the tooth is displaced *totally out* of its socket. Clinically, the socket is found empty or filled with a coagulum.

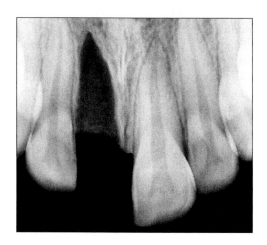

RADIOGRAPHIC APPEARANCE

The socket is empty; fracture lines in the socket may be present.

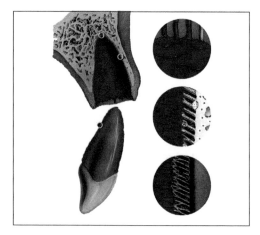

BIOLOGICAL CONSIDERATIONS AND TREATMENT PRINCIPLES

Immediately after injury, the PDL and pulp of the avulsed tooth begin to suffer ischemic injury, which is soon aggravated by drying, exposure to bacteria or chemical irritants. These events can kill PDL and pulpal cells even after a short extra-alveolar period.[111] Treatment outcome is strongly dependent on the length of the dry extra-alveolar time period and the storage media used.[111] If the extra-alveolar period is less than 1 hour, complete or partial PDL healing is possible. However, total PDL death can be expected after more than 1 hour of drying (delayed replantation); and progressive root resorption will be the result.[111] While some might argue that due to the certainty of resorption in replanting teeth with more than 1 hour extra-alveolar exposure, such teeth should not be replanted, it is important to consider that with techniques such as decoronation, delayed replantation of teeth in children can be beneficial in order to save and maintain the alveolar growth in the region (see page 68). In patients with fully formed teeth, delayed replantation can allow for many years of good service.[111]

Traumatic Dental Injuries: A Manual, Third Edition © J.O. Andreasen, L.K. Bakland, M.T. Flores, F.M. Andreasen and L. Andersson
Published 2011 by Blackwell Publishing Ltd

FIRST AID FOR AVULSED TEETH

Dentists should always be prepared to give appropriate advice to the public about first aid for avulsed teeth.[112] An avulsed permanent tooth is one of the few real emergency situations in dentistry. Public awareness needs to be increased, and health care professionals, parents and teachers should receive information on how to proceed following these severe, unexpected injuries. Instructions can be given by telephone to parents when an emergency occurs. If a tooth has been avulsed, make sure it is a permanent tooth (primary teeth should not be replanted).[112]

When a tooth has been knocked out:

- Keep the patient calm.
- Find the tooth and pick it up by the crown (the white part). Avoid touching the root.

- If the tooth is dirty, wash it briefly (10 seconds) under cold running water and then reposition it. Try to encourage the patient/parent to replant the tooth. Bite on a handkerchief to hold it in position.
- If it is not possible to reposition the tooth, place the tooth in a suitable storage medium, e.g. a glass of milk or a special storage media for avulsed teeth, if available. The tooth can also be transported in the mouth, keeping it between the molars and the inside of the cheek. Avoid storage in water.
- Seek emergency dental treatment immediately.

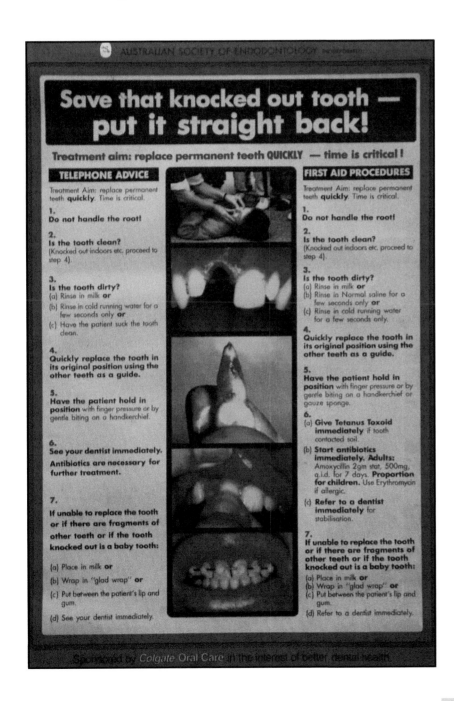

TREATMENT SCENARIOS

The following situations may preclude replantation of an avulsed tooth: age of the patient (primary tooth); extensive carious destruction of the tooth; extensive loss of marginal periodontal support; medically compromised patients (e.g. infectious endocarditis, immunosuppressive treatment).

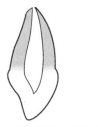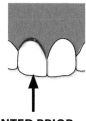

TOOTH REPLANTED PRIOR TO ARRIVAL

CLOSED APEX: TOOTH REPLANTED PRIOR TO THE PATIENT'S ARRIVAL AT THE CLINIC

- Leave the tooth in place.
- Clean the area with water spray, saline, or chlorhexidine.
- Suture gingival lacerations, if present.
- Verify normal position of the replanted tooth both clinically and radiographically.
- Apply a flexible splint for up to 2 weeks.
- Administer systemic antibiotics.

Please remember to read the sections on antibiotics, patient information and follow-up

CLOSED APEX: EXTRAORAL DRY TIME LESS THAN 60 MIN. THE TOOTH HAS BEEN KEPT IN PHYSIOLOGIC STORAGE MEDIA

Physiologic media include Hank's balanced salt solution, milk, physiologic saline or saliva.

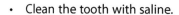

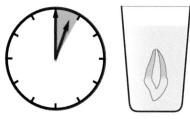

DRY TIME LESS THAN 60 MIN

- Clean the tooth with saline.
- Irrigate the socket with saline.
- Examine the alveolar socket. If there is a fracture of the socket wall, reposition it with a suitable instrument.
- Replant the tooth with gentle pressure. Do *not* use force!
- Suture gingival lacerations, if present.
- Verify normal position of the replanted tooth both clinically and radiographically.
- Apply a flexible splint for up to 2 weeks.
- Administer systemic antibiotics.

Please remember to read the sections on antibiotics, patient information and follow-up

CLOSED APEX: EXTRAORAL DRY TIME EXCEEDING 60 MIN. OR LONG STORAGE IN NON-PHYSIOLOGIC MEDIA

Delayed replantation has a poor long-term prognosis. The periodontal ligament will be necrotic and cannot be expected to heal. The goal in doing delayed replantation is to promote alveolar bone growth to encapsulate the replanted tooth. The expected outcome is ankylosis and resorption of the root. In children below the age of 15, when ankylosis occurs, and when infraposition of the tooth crown is more than 1 mm, it is recommended to perform decoronation to preserve the contour of the alveolar ridge (see page 68). Before replantation the tooth should be placed in 2% sodium fluoride solution, a treatment which slows subsequent resorption.[113]

- Remove attached necrotic soft tissue with gauze.
- Root canal treatment can be performed prior to replantation, or it can be done 7–10 days later.
- Immerse the tooth in a 2% sodium fluoride solution for 20 min.
- Irrigate the socket with saline.
- Examine the alveolar socket. If there is a fracture of the socket wall, reposition it with a suitable instrument.
- Replant the tooth with gentle pressure.
- Suture gingival lacerations, if present.
- Verify normal position of the replanted tooth clinically and radiographically.
- Stabilize the tooth for 4 weeks using a flexible splint.
- Administer systemic antibiotics.

Please remember to read the sections on antibiotics, patient information and follow-up

DRY TIME EXCEEDING 60 MIN

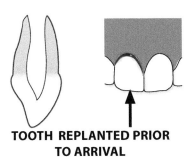

TOOTH REPLANTED PRIOR TO ARRIVAL

OPEN APEX: TOOTH REPLANTED PRIOR TO THE PATIENTS ARRIVAL AT THE CLINIC

- Leave the tooth in place.
- Clean the area with water spray, saline, or chlorhexidine.
- Suture gingival laceration, if present.
- Verify normal position of the replanted tooth both clinically and radiographically.
- Apply a flexible splint for up to 2 weeks.
- Administer systemic antibiotics.

Please remember to read the sections on antibiotics, patient information and follow-up

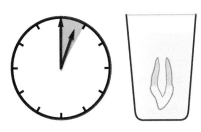

DRY TIME LESS THAN 60 MIN

OPEN APEX: EXTRAORAL DRY TIME LESS THAN 60 MIN. THE TOOTH HAS BEEN KEPT IN PHYSIOLOGIC STORAGE MEDIA

Physiologic media include Hank's balanced salt solution, milk, physiologic saline or saliva.

- Clean the tooth with saline.
- Irrigate the socket with saline.
- If available, cover the root surface with minocycline hydrochloride microspheres before replanting the tooth or soak it in a doxycycline solution (1 mg/20 ml saline).[114–118]
- Examine the alveolar socket. If there is a fracture of the socket wall, reposition it with a suitable instrument.
- Replant the tooth with gentle pressure. Do *not* use force!
- Suture gingival lacerations, especially in the cervical area.
- Verify normal position of the replanted tooth clinically and radiographically.
- Apply a flexible splint for up to 2 weeks.
- Administer systemic antibiotics.

Please remember to read the sections on antibiotics, patient information and follow-up

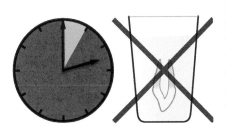

DRY TIME EXCEEDING 60 MIN

OPEN APEX: EXTRAORAL DRY TIME EXCEEDING 60 MIN. OR LONGER STORAGE IN NON-PHYSIOLOGIC MEDIA

Delayed replantation has a poor long-term prognosis. The periodontal ligament will be necrotic and not expected to heal. The goal in doing delayed replantation of immature teeth in children is to maintain alveolar ridge contour. The eventual outcome is expected to be ankylosis and resorption of the root. It is important to recognize that if delayed replantation is done in a child, future treatment planning must include taking into account the expected tooth ankylosis and the effect of ankylosis on the alveolar ridge development. When ankylosis occurs, and when the infraposition of the tooth crown is more than 1 mm, it is recommended to perform decoronation to preserve the contour of the alveolar ridge (see page 68).

- Remove attached necrotic soft tissue with gauze.
- Root canal treatment can be performed prior to replantation through the open apex.
- Immerse the tooth in a 2% sodium fluoride solution for 20 min.
- Irrigate the socket with saline.
- Examine the alveolar socket. If there is a fracture of the socket wall, reposition it with a suitable instrument.
- Replant the tooth with gentle pressure.
- Suture gingival lacerations, if present.
- Verify normal position of the replanted tooth clinically and radiographically.
- Stabilize the tooth for 4 weeks using a flexible splint.
- Administer systemic antibiotics.

Please remember to read the sections on antibiotics, patient information and follow-up

ANTIBIOTICS

The value of systemic administration of antibiotics after replantation of avulsed teeth is still questionable as clinical studies have not demonstrated its value.[111] Animal studies have, however, usually shown some positive effect upon both PDL healing and pulp healing when administrated topically.[115–120] Tetracycline is the first choice (doxycycline 2 times per day for 7 days at appropriate dose for patient age and weight).[119] The risk of discoloration of permanent teeth must be considered before systemic administration of tetracycline in young patients (in many countries tetracycline is not recommended for patients under 12 years of age). In young patients phenoxymethyl penicillin (Pen V), at an appropriate dosage for age and weight, is an alternative to tetracycline.[112]

TETANUS PROPHYLAXIS

If the avulsed tooth has contacted soil, and if tetanus coverage is uncertain, refer to a physician for evaluation and need for a tetanus booster.

PATIENT INSTRUCTIONS

- Soft food for up to 2 weeks.
- Brush teeth with a soft toothbrush after each meal.
- Use a chlorhexidine (0.1%) mouth rinse twice a day for 1 week.

ENDODONTIC CONSIDERATIONS

Due to the associated pulp and PDL injuries, the risk of root resorption is great. Consequently, the following endodontic treatment rules are suggested based on present experimental and clinical studies,[121,122] as well as recommended guidelines.[112]

TEETH WITH CLOSED APICES

Pulp revascularization is not likely to occur; and as a prophylactic measure against development of root resorption the pulp should be extirpated 7–10 days after replantation.[111] Calcium hydroxide is placed in the root canal and the tooth should be permanently root filled with gutta percha and a sealer after 2–4 weeks.

TEETH WITH OPEN APICES

Pulp revascularization is possible although relatively rare. Pulp necrosis is usually evident after 2–4 weeks and presents with periapical rarefaction with or without signs of inflammatory root resorption.[111] As soon as the diagnosis of pulp necrosis has been made, the pulp should be extirpated and the root canal biomechanically cleansed and medicated with calcium hydroxide. This technique is described on page 64.

FOLLOW-UP

The splint is removed after 2 weeks, or 4 weeks if the PDL has been removed. Please view the individual instructions for the six listed healing scenarios as regards length of splinting. If pulpal revascularization is not to be expected (teeth with closed apices), the pulp is extirpated prior to splint removal and calcium hydroxide is placed in the root canal as an interim dressing. Completion of the root canal treatment is described on page 64. In all cases, a radiographic control should be made once a week during the first month. At these times, signs of infection-related resorption may be present, which will dictate pulpal extirpation, and also in teeth with incomplete root formation.[111] Further radiographic and clinical controls should be made after 3 months, 6 months and then yearly for 5 years at which time ankylosis, if it is going to occur, can usually be demonstrated.[121–145] Pulpal and periodontal healing have been found to be mainly dependent on three factors:[121–145]

- Length of extra-alveolar storage.
- Extra-alveolar storage medium.
- Stage of root development.

In the graphs on page 53, the survival rates of pulp, periodontal ligament and tooth survival are presented as they relate to the above-mentioned factors.[123–127]

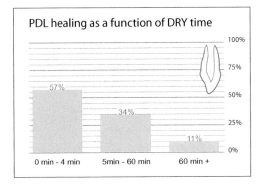

Pulp healing as a function of DRY time

0 min - 4 min: 48%
5min - 60 min: 27%
60 min +: 11%

EXPECTED OUTCOME: PULP

The healing potential of the pulp appears to be related to the length of the dry extra-alveolar storage period.[124]

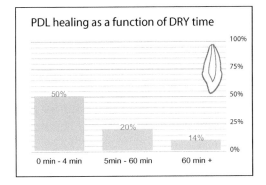

PDL healing as a function of DRY time

0 min - 4 min: 57%
5min - 60 min: 34%
60 min +: 11%

EXPECTED OUTCOME: PDL

Healing appears to be strongly related to the length of the dry and the wet extra-alveolar storage period for teeth with incomplete root formation.[126]

PDL healing as a function of DRY time

0 min - 4 min: 50%
5min - 60 min: 20%
60 min +: 14%

EXPECTED OUTCOME: PDL

Healing appears to be strongly related to the length of the dry extra-alveolar storage period for teeth with complete root formation.[126]

NOTES

_____
_____
_____
_____
_____
_____
_____
_____
_____
_____
_____

Injuries to the Primary Dentition

OBJECTIVES

1 Recognize the various trauma entities in the primary dentition.

2 Recognize the risk of concomitant trauma to the permanent dentition.

3 Determine treatment options that will reduce the risk of disturbances in development of the permanent dentition.

4 Determine risk profile for primary tooth trauma that presents a significant risk for the permanent succedaneous dentition.

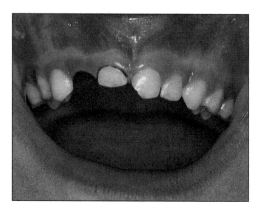

DESCRIPTION AND CLINICAL APPEARANCE

These traumas result in loss of tooth substance or displacement of primary teeth.

The clinical appearance of trauma in the primary dentition is similar to that in the permanent dentition. This figure illustrates avulsion (right lateral primary incisor), intrusion (right central primary incisor) and an uncomplicated crown fracture (left central primary incisor).

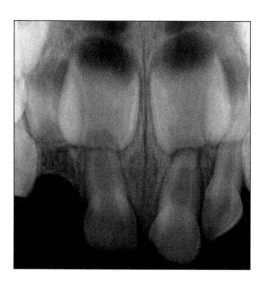

RADIOGRAPHIC APPEARANCE

It shows the degree of development of the primary tooth and its permanent successor and the relationship between the two. However, an important goal in the radiographic examination is to determine whether the primary tooth has invaded the follicle of the developing subjacent succedaneous tooth. The radiographic presentation here illustrates the clinical situation shown above.

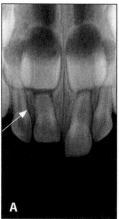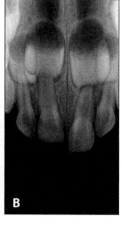

RADIOGRAPHIC TECHNIQUE FOR DETERMINING INVASION OF THE FOLLICLE

A radiograph of the anterior region should include all anterior teeth, with the jaw midline corresponding to the midline of the radiographic film. A foreshortened image of the luxated tooth indicates that the primary root apex has been forced labially (arrow), away from the follicle (Figure A).[146] An elongated image suggests displacement in the opposite direction, and thus a risk for invasion into the developing tooth follicle (Figure B). The developing teeth should appear symmetric (Figure A). If the distance between the incisal edge and the mineralization front of the developing tooth is less on the injured side than on the non-injured side (Figure B), there is a significant risk that the intruded primary tooth has displaced the developing permanent tooth germ. This finding indicates immediate removal of the primary tooth.

Traumatic Dental Injuries: A Manual, Third Edition   © J.O. Andreasen, L.K. Bakland, M.T. Flores, F.M. Andreasen and L. Andersson
Published 2011 by Blackwell Publishing Ltd

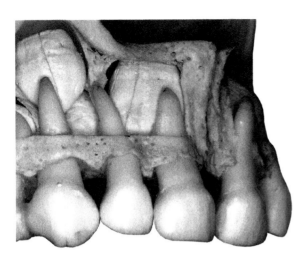

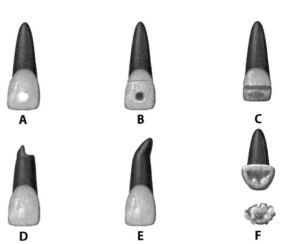

BIOLOGICAL CONSIDERATIONS

The very close proximity of the developing permanent successors to the apices of the primary teeth makes the transmission of traumatic forces from luxation injuries a very likely event.[146,147]

Moreover, inflammation related to pulpal complications in the displaced primary tooth may add further injury.[147] In fact, approximately one-half of all primary tooth injuries result in more or less severe disturbances in permanent tooth development. These disturbances range from mineralization disturbances to complete malformation of the tooth germ, as illustrated: Figure A, white or yellow enamel opacity; Figure B, yellow–brown enamel opacity with or without hypoplasia; Figure C, yellow–brown enamel opacity with circumferential hypoplasia; Figure D, partial arrest of root formation; Figure E, root dilacerations; and Figure F, root angulation and odontoma-like malformation.

TREATMENT PRINCIPLES

The primary goal is to optimize periodontal and pulpal healing in the primary dentition provided that no further injury is transmitted to the developing permanent successors.[146,148]

Recent animal studies indicate that similar pulpal and periodontal healing responses to acute dental traumas are found in both dentitions.[146] Concerning transmission of trauma to the developing successor, the major effect seems to originate from the initial trauma, with little effect from repositioning or extraction of the displaced primary tooth.[147] One exception, however, is when the primary tooth is intruded directly into the follicle and immediate extraction of the primary tooth appears to be the treatment of choice.[147]

Periapical infection may occur due to an infected pulp necrosis in the primary tooth. This indicates extraction of the primary tooth to avoid a known long-term effect of inflammation on mineralization of the permanent tooth germ.[147] In selected cases endodontic treatment may be chosen.

TREATMENT

The management of traumatic injuries to primary teeth differs from treatment of permanent teeth.[146] Three factors have a major influence on the selection of treatment for injured primary teeth:

- The relatively short period primary teeth are in function in the child's mouth.
- The close proximity of the root of the primary tooth to its developing permanent successor.
- The difficulty of gaining the child's compliance.

Crown fractures

Uncomplicated fractures are treated by smoothing of sharp edges. If possible the tooth can be restored with glass ionomer filling material or composite. Teeth with exposed pulps are usually extracted if patient cooperation is a problem. In cooperative children pulp capping or pulpotomy may be performed.[146]

Crown-root fractures

Extraction is recommended.[146] Care must be taken to prevent trauma to the subjacent tooth bud.[146,148]

Root fractures

Root fractures with minimal displacement of the coronal fragment can be left untreated and will resorb at the expected time. If the coronal fragment is displaced, extract only that fragment. The apical fragment can be left for physiological resoption.[146,148]

Displaced coronal fragments can be repositioned. However, splinting is generally neither possible nor necessary. Should pulp necrosis occur, the coronal fragment should be extracted while the apical fragment is left to resorb physiologically. The permanent tooth eruption will not be affected.[146]

Concussion and subluxation

Observation.[146,148]

Extrusion

Treatment decisions are based on the degree of displacement, mobility, root formation and the ability of the child to cope with the emergency situation. For minor extrusion (<3 mm) in an immature developing tooth, careful repositioning or leaving the tooth for spontaneous alignment are acceptable treatment options. Extraction is the treatment of choice for severe extrusion in a fully formed primary tooth.[148]

Lateral luxation

Most laterally luxated teeth are displaced with the crowns in a palatal lingual direction. This indicates that the apex is displaced away from the permanent tooth germ. If there is no occlusal interference, the tooth should be allowed to reposition spontaneously.[146,148] When there is occlusal interference, with the use of local anesthesia, the tooth can be gently repositioned by combined labial and palatal pressure. In severe displacement, when the crown is dislocated in a labial direction, extraction is the treatment of choice. If there is minor occlusal interference, slight grinding is indicated.[148]

Intrusion

Due to the labial curvature of the apex, most intruded teeth are displaced through the labial bone plate. These teeth can, therefore, be left to re-erupt spontaneously. A few teeth are intruded directly into the developing tooth germ and should be removed.[146]

Avulsion

A radiographic examination is essential to ensure that the missing tooth is not intruded. Avulsed primary teeth should not be replanted.[146]

Alveolar fracture

Reposition any displaced segment and then splint. General anesthesia is often indicated. Monitor teeth in fracture line.[148]

FOLLOW-UP

Control visits are necessary to diagnose healing complications. These are primarily pulpal complications related to infected pulp necrosis following luxation injuries, and are related to the type of luxation.[146–149] Post-trauma control visits should be performed 1 week, 3–4 weeks, 6–8 weeks, 6 months and 1 year after injury. In cases of complicated trauma (intrusions and avulsions), a further radiographic control is indicated just before eruption of the permanent successor to register any disturbances in tooth development or eruption.

EXPECTED OUTCOME

The long-term prognosis should include the fate of the injured primary tooth and that of the permanent successor. The risk of pulp necrosis in the primary dentition appears to be related to the type of luxation injury and the stage of root development at the time of injury.[150–158] The risk of disturbances in the permanent dentition appears also to be related to the type of luxation injury and the age of the patient (see following pages).[150–158]

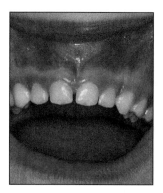 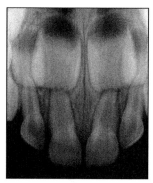 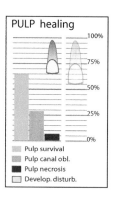

CONCUSSION

Pulp healing is frequent.[149] There are presently no data on the frequency of developmental disturbances in the permanent dentition.

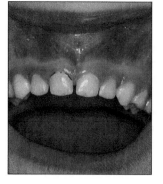 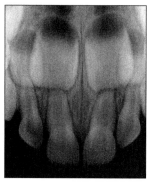 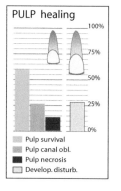

SUBLUXATION

Pulp healing is frequent. Complications in the permanent dentition are relatively rare and usually consist of enamel discoloration.[149,151]

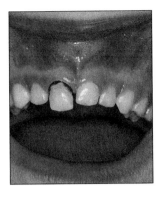
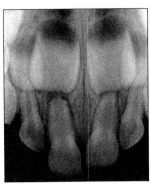
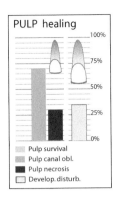

PULP healing

100%
75%
50%
25%
0%

☐ Pulp survival
☐ Pulp canal obl.
■ Pulp necrosis
☐ Develop. disturb.

EXTRUSION

Pulp healing is dependent upon stage of root development. There is moderate risk of complications to the permanent dentition.[147]

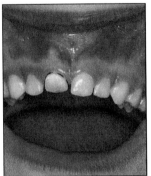
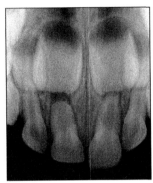
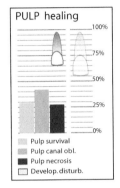

PULP healing

100%
75%
50%
25%
0%

☐ Pulp survival
☐ Pulp canal obl.
■ Pulp necrosis
☐ Develop. disturb.

LATERAL LUXATION

Pulp healing is dependent on the stage of root development.[146] There is presently no information about the risk of developmental changes in the permanent dentition.

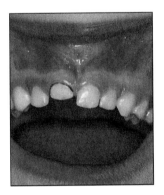
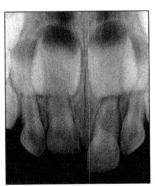
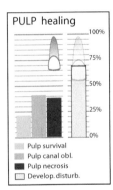

PULP healing

100%
75%
50%
25%
0%

☐ Pulp survival
☐ Pulp canal obl.
■ Pulp necrosis
☐ Develop. disturb.

INTRUSION

Pulp necrosis is frequent, as are complications in the permanent dentition.[147]

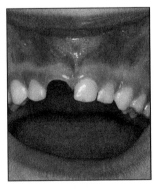
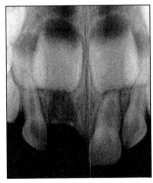
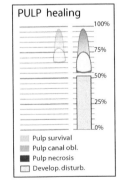

PULP healing

100%
75%
50%
25%
0%

☐ Pulp survival
☐ Pulp canal obl.
■ Pulp necrosis
☐ Develop. disturb.

AVULSION

Complications in the permanent dentition are frequent.[147]

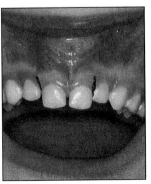
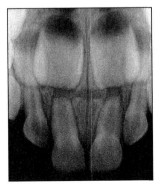
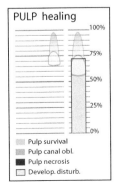

PULP healing

100%
75%
50%
25%
0%

☐ Pulp survival
☐ Pulp canal obl.
■ Pulp necrosis
☐ Develop. disturb.

FRACTURE OF THE ALVEOLAR PROCESS

Complications in the permanent dentition are frequent.[147]

Soft Tissue Injuries

DESCRIPTION AND CLINICAL APPEARANCE

Traumatic injuries to teeth are often associated with injuries to various soft tissue areas including oral mucosa, lips and facial skin. Foreign material (dirt, asphalt and even tooth fragments) may be embedded in the soft tissue wound areas. Careful evaluation of these areas of trauma is essential during the initial injury examination. The following are the types of soft tissue injuries one might encounter in an accident victim.[159]

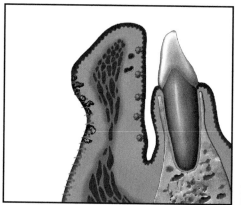 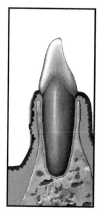

ABRASION OF SKIN, MUCOSA AND GINGIVA

A superficial wound produced by rubbing and scraping of the mucosa or skin leaving a raw, bleeding surface which, however, remains partly covered with epithelium. The presence of epithelium is important as healing consists of proliferation of a new epithelial cover from the remaining basal layers of the epithelium and appendices.[159]

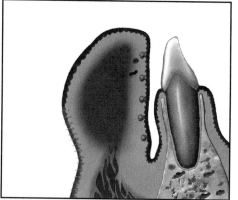 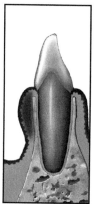

CONTUSION OF SKIN, MUCOSA AND GINGIVA

A bruise without a break in the skin or mucosa represented as a subcutaneous or submucosal tissue hemorrhage. A contusion may be isolated to soft tissue or indicate an underlying bone fracture.[159]

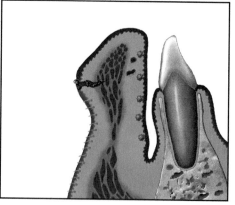 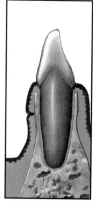

SUPERFICIAL LACERATION OF SKIN, MUCOSA OR GINGIVA

A wound in the skin or mucosa penetrating into the soft tissue. Lacerations will disrupt blood vessels, nerves and sometimes muscles, hair follicles and salivary glands. The most frequently affected sites are lips, oral mucosa and gingiva. More seldom the tongue is involved.[159]

Traumatic Dental Injuries: A Manual, Third Edition   © J.O. Andreasen, L.K. Bakland, M.T. Flores, F.M. Andreasen and L. Andersson
Published 2011 by Blackwell Publishing Ltd

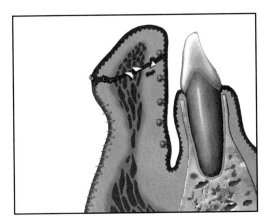

PENETRATING LIP WOUNDS

In these types of lacerations, which penetrate from skin to mucosa, the presence of foreign bodies are very common.[159]

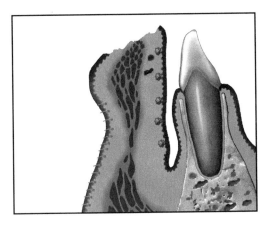

AVULSION OF SKIN, MUCOSA AND GINGIVA

Tissue avulsion (loss of tissue) are rare but seen in association with bite injuries or as a result of a very deep and extended abrasion.[159]

TREATMENT PRINCIPLES FOR SOFT TISSUE WOUNDS

MECHANICAL MANIPULATION OF THE WOUND

An important general principle is the need for meticulous cleansing and debridement of oral and cutaneous wounds, as presence of bacteria and especially foreign bodies increases the risk of healing complications. Secondly, wound approximation using tension-free sutures is essential for rapid healing.[160–173]

ANTIBIOTICS AND TETANUS PROPHYLAXIS TREATMENT

A controversial issue has been use of antibiotics as part of treatment for soft tissue injuries; no reliable randomized studies in regard to oral wounds have been published.[169] The few studies reported seem to indicate that superficial lacerations do not benefit from antibiotic treatment,[169,170] whereas penetrating lip lesions possibly need antibiotic coverage to lower the risk of inflammatory complications.[161] The current recommendations for using antibiotics appear to be:

ANTIBIOTIC PROPHYLAXIS

Antibiotics should be given in the following situations:
- Heavily contaminated wound.
- Compromised wound cleansing, e.g. restricted vascularity of the injured tissue.
- Delayed treatment > 24 hours.
- Injuries penetrating through the lip or the cheek.
- Human and animal bite wounds.
- Simultaneous extensive bone surgery such as open reduction of a bone fracture.
- When the general defense system of the patient is compromised, e.g. insulin-dependent diabetes and immunocompromised patients.
- Patients with risk of infective endocarditis such as cardiac valves or cardiac reconstruction, valvar dysfunction/malformation or previous endocarditis. The recommendations may vary for different countries. Read more about current recommendations for infective endocarditis from the American Heart Association (www.americanheart.org).

TETANUS PROPHYLAXIS

In cases of contaminated wounds, tetanus prophylaxis should be considered. Check if the patient is immunized. If more than 5 years since last immunization have elapsed, a booster dose should be considered.

TREATMENT

ABRASIONS AND CONTUSIONS

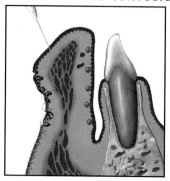

Apply local anesthesia as topical and/or regional injection.

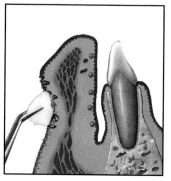

Rinse the abrasion with saline. Use gauze swabs or a soft tooth brush.

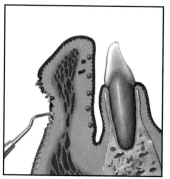

Remove all foreign bodies with a small excavator or a surgical scalpel. Removal of all foreign bodies is essential for good healing. Failure to do so may result in permanent tattooing and scarring. Intraoral abrasions do not have to be treated apart from removal of foreign bodies.

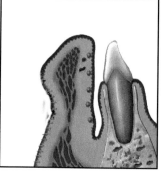

In case of contusions perform a radiographic examination to examine for bone fractures, which may require separate treatment. No treatment is necessary for contusions when the injury is limited to soft tissue. Make sure that there is no ongoing deep bleeding; if a swelling is located in the floor of the mouth there may be a risk of blocking the airway. Such patients need to be observed for several hours.

NON-PENETRATING LACERATIONS

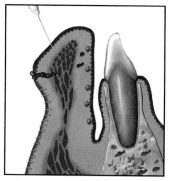

Administer local or regional anesthesia.

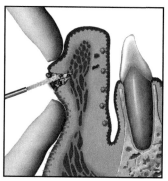

Open up the wound and inspect it for the presence of foreign bodies. In the case of deep wounds supplement with a radiographic examination (see penetrating lip lesions).

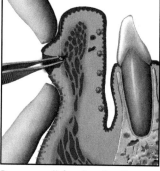

Remove all foreign bodies during the emergency phase of treatment to prevent infection and disfiguring scarring or tattooing of the skin. Use a syringe with saline under high pressure or gauze swabs soaked in saline. Foreign bodies can be removed with a small spoon-shaped excavator.

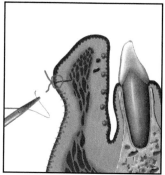

Suture with single interrupted sutures in the oral mucosa and gingiva. Use either absorbable or non-absorbable suture material in sizes 4-0 to 5-0 for intraoral sutures. For suturing skin, a thinner suture, size 6-0, is preferable. When suturing lip wounds, special attention must be paid to carefully approximate the transition of skin to mucosa as any inaccuracy in wound closure will result in poor esthetic healing. With deep lacerations, suturing in layers is indicated. Adhesive tape/strips may be used to relieve tension across the wound.

PENETRATING LACERATIONS OF THE LIP

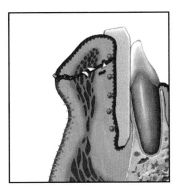 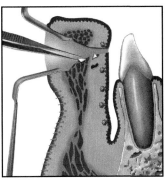 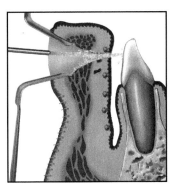 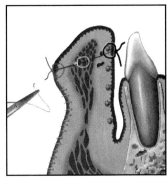

In these cases a radiographic examination is always indicated due to the risk of foreign bodies. Place a film between the lip and the alveolar process and use an exposure of 25% of the dose for a normal intraoral radiograph.

Administer a local or regional anesthetic and open the wound with finger pressure or with wound retractors. Look for any foreign bodies that may have showed on the radiograph. Count the number of foreign bodies removed and compare these numbers and positions with the radiographic appearances.

Next, use a syringe with saline under high pressure supplemented with gauze swabs soaked in saline to further clean the wound.

Suture the oral lesion with interrupted sutures. Use either absorbable or non-absorbable sutures in sizes 4.0 or 5.0.
Place a few absorbable deep sutures in the musculature. Finish suturing the skin by using interrupted non-absorbable sutures size 6.0 separated with a distance of 4 mm. Adhesive tape/strips may be used to relieve the tension across the wound.

SOFT TISSUE AVULSION

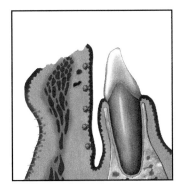

In cases of soft tissue avulsion, administer local anesthesia and clean the wound. Small defects can be left for spontaneous healing. With extensive tissue loss, excision and primary closure using flaps and grafts may be necessary.

Splinting

The application of a splint is indicated in all cases where repositioning has been performed after a luxation or avulsion injury and root or alveolar bone fracture.[174] Several studies have shown that a flexible splint may optimize pulp and PDL healing.[175–187] The flexibility of various splint types has been tested in in-vitro situations.[178–186] Two general types of splint exist in this category: a flexible temporization material splint and a flexible wire/fiber composite splint.

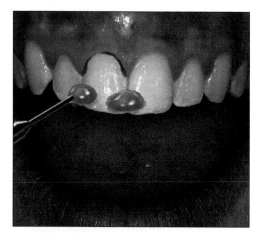

ETCHING ENAMEL

The incisal one-third of the labial aspect of enamel on the injured and adjacent teeth is acid-etched (30 seconds) with phosphoric acid gel.

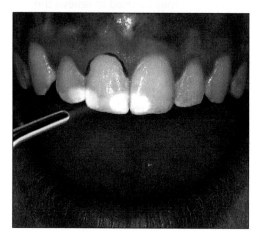

RINSING AND DRYING ENAMEL

The etchant is removed with a 20-second water spray and the enamel dried with a stream of compressed air; the etched enamel has a matte, chalky appearance. The teeth are isolated with gauze sponges labially and palatally. Hemostasis can be achieved by compressing these sponges with firm finger pressure.

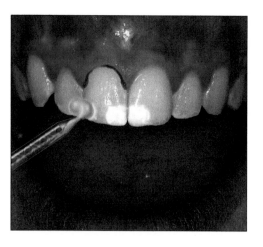

FLEXIBLE TEMPORIZATION MATERIAL SPLINT

The splinting material is applied in a thin layer. A temporization material (e.g. Protemp®, Luxatemp®, Isotemp®, Provipond®, Structure®, Acrytemp®) is used, whereby a semi-rigid splint is created. During polymerization of the splinting material, the patient may occlude to ensure correct repositioning of the tooth. Keep the splint away from the gingiva to permit optimal oral hygiene.

Traumatic Dental Injuries: A Manual, Third Edition   © J.O. Andreasen, L.K. Bakland, M.T. Flores, F.M. Andreasen and L. Andersson
Published 2011 by Blackwell Publishing Ltd

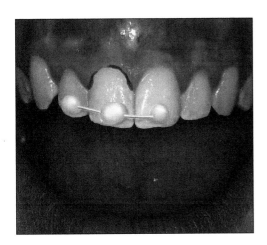

FLEXIBLE WIRE/FIBER COMPOSITE SPLINT

There are a number of wire/fiber systems on the market where the flexibility of the splint is ensured by various means. These include glass fiber (Kevlar®), nylon, orthodontic wire, twist flex wire, fiber (Ribbond®) and titanium plates.

It is important that the reinforcing wires/fibers are placed inside the composite material for labial bonding of the injured and adjacent teeth.

Bonded orthodontic brackets can also be used. This form of splinting has the advantage in multiple tooth injuries that the various splinting periods can be respected without removing the splint.

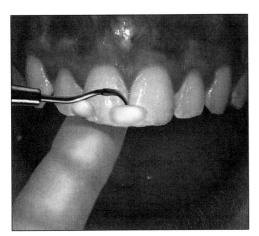

REMOVING A TEMPORIZATION MATERIAL SPLINT

At the end of the fixation period, the splint is removed with either a scaler or a fissure bur. The enamel is then lightly polished to re-establish a smooth surface.

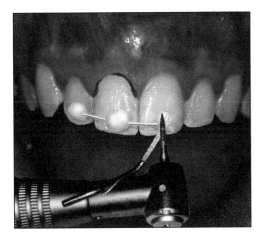

REMOVING A FLEXIBLE WIRE/FIBER COMPOSITE SPLINT

The composite material is removed with a bur and the enamel is then polished.

SPLINTING TIMES

Subluxation	2 weeks
Extrusive luxation	2 weeks
Avulsion	2 weeks
Lateral luxation	4 weeks
Root fracture (apical and middle third)	4 weeks
Alveolar bone fracture	4 weeks
Root fracture (cervical third)	4 months

Endodontic Considerations in Dental Trauma

OBJECTIVES

1. Recognize differences in caries and trauma-related pulp pathosis.
2. Define treatment goals.
3. Determine the effects of bacteria on healing events after trauma.
4. Recognize how resorption processes may interfere with the endodontic procedures.
5. Recognize the endodontic problems of exposed vital pulps in teeth with open and closed apices.
6. Recognize the endodontic problems of necrotic pulps in teeth with root fractures.
7. Recognize the endodontic problems of teeth with associated external root resorption.

PULP AND PERIODONTAL LIGAMENT PATHOSIS FOLLOWING DENTAL CARIES AND DENTAL TRAUMA

There appears to be major differences in etiology and pathogenesis of pulp pathosis related to caries progression and dental trauma.[188, 189] The main therapeutic problem in caries-related infected pulp necrosis appears to be control of bacteria in the pulp canal. Obturation of the root canal is for the most part an uncomplicated procedure in teeth with fully developed roots. In cases of trauma-related pulp necrosis (see page 22), which frequently occur in developing teeth with open apices, problems in root canal obturation, however, are often encountered. Furthermore, infection-related external root resorption (see page 24) cannot be arrested without proper disinfection of the root canal and dentinal tubules. Finally, due to its remodeling character, ankylosis can expose dentinal tubules, resulting in direct or indirect exposure of the potentially contaminated root canal content.

PROBLEMS OF PULP NECROSIS AND DEVELOPING ROOT FORMATION: TREATMENT OBJECTIVES

An open apex represents a major obstacle in disinfecting and obturating the root canal. Experimental and clinical studies have shown that bacteria are located in the necrotic pulp and surrounding dentinal tubules (Figure A). Removal of necrotic pulp tissue and disinfection of the root canal will lead to healing processes that in most cases result in closure of the apical area by a hard tissue barrier formed by cementoblasts. In rare cases where the Hertwig's epithelial root sheath has survived, dentin and cementum may be formed resulting in additional root length (apexogenesis). Due to the frequently weakened structure of the immature root, treatment approaches should be selected which do not further weaken the tooth (i.e. extensive root canal filing or extensive chemical treatment of the canal [e.g. prolonged treatment with calcium hydroxide]), which can lead to spontaneous cervical root fracture.

PROBLEMS WITH INFECTION-RELATED ROOT RESORPTION

The presence of infection-related root resorption cavities on the root surface represents a significant threat to the prognosis of the endodontic procedure (Figure B). Unless all bacteria are permanently removed or inactivated in the root canal as well as the dentinal tubules, resorption may progress. If, however, bacteria are removed or inactivated, healing will take place with a new periodontal ligament inserted into newly formed cementum, or an ankylosis (in case of extensive resorption cavities).

PROBLEMS OF ANKYLOSIS-RELATED RESORPTION

Due to the inherently progressive nature of the ankylotic process (see page 25), where dentinal tubules may be exposed by osteoclastic activity, effective root canal obturation is essential. Furthermore, a bacteria-tight seal must be created at the entrance of the root canal. Unless these steps are taken, a slowly progressive ankylosis-related resorption may change to a rapidly invading infection-related resorption.

TIME RELATION OF VARIOUS PROPERTIES OF CALCIUM HYDROXIDE

For decades, calcium hydroxide has been known to be a very effective medication in the treatment of pulpal and periodontal complications following injury. This is primarily related to simultaneous disinfection of pulp tissue and the capacity to initiate hard tissue healing. Knowledge about the time relationship of these effects is necessary for its proper use. Calcium hydroxide is known to have a strong proteolytic effect.[190] Thus, most pulp remnants will be completely dissolved within 1 week. However, the same proteolytic effect apparently also affects the circumpulpal dentin, resulting over time (months) in its weakening.[191] This is possibly the

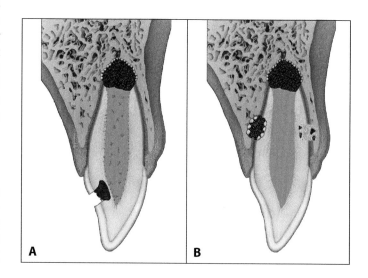

A   B

Traumatic Dental Injuries: A Manual, Third Edition   © J.O. Andreasen, L.K. Bakland, M.T. Flores, F.M. Andreasen and L. Andersson
Published 2011 by Blackwell Publishing Ltd

explanation for the occurrence of cervical root fractures in more than half of the endodontically treated teeth with immature root formation subjected to long-term (> 1 month) calcium hydroxide placement.[192] The use of calcium hydroxide should therefore be limited to a few weeks.

PULP NECROSIS WITH OR WITHOUT INFECTION-RELATED RESORPTION: COMPLETED ROOT FORMATION

After pulp extirpation, calcium hydroxide is used as an interim root canal dressing to disinfect the root canal and dentinal

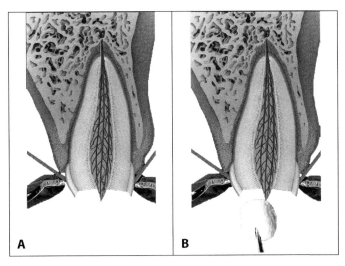

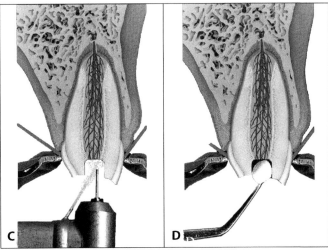

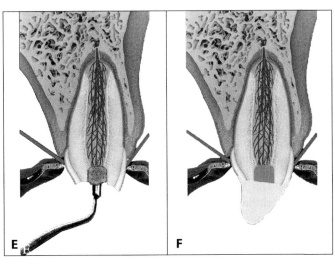

tubules, to dissolve necrotic pulp remnants and to arrest osteoclastic activity on the external root surface. After 2 weeks, the root canal space is obturated with gutta percha and sealer. It is important to create a bacteria-tight seal in the cervical root canal region to prevent reactivation of resorption processes or periapical inflammation.

TREATMENT OF TRAUMATIC DENTAL INJURIES USING MINERAL TRIOXIDE AGGREGATE

Mineral trioxide aggregate (MTA; ProRoot MTA®, Root Canal Repair Material Dentsply Tulsa Dental, Tulsa, OK, USA) has been shown to be a very useful dental material for the treatment of many conditions, including traumatic dental injuries.[193–206] The material is currently used in vital pulp therapy, as apical plugs in teeth with open apices, and to provide a barrier at the site of root fractures when the coronal pulp in such teeth must be extirpated and replaced with a filling material.[195–206]

PULP CAPPING AND PULPOTOMY

Pulp capping and pulpotomy are procedures aimed at protecting the vital pulp from bacterial invasion and, in young teeth, allow for continued root development. Calcium hydroxide has been the most commonly used agent, in combination with restorative materials, for achieving these goals. MTA has several advantages over calcium hydroxide: it provides protection against bacterial penetration, does not disintegrate over time, and after setting provides a hard surface against which other dental materials can be placed.[196–200] Pulp capping with calcium hydroxide is described on page 30. The use of MTA in connection with pulpotomy is described in the following.

(Figure A) Isolate the tooth with a rubber dam after administering local anesthesia.

(Figure B) Disinfect the exposed dentin and pulp with either sodium hypochlorite or Peridex®.

(Figure C) Remove pulp and surrounding dentin to a depth of 2 mm from the level of exposure, using a round diamond bur and water or saline spray.

(Figure D) Place a saline-moistened cotton pellet onto the pulpal wound until bleeding has ceased, or nearly so. An effective method for controlling bleeding is to place a cotton pellet moistened with sodium hypochlorite solution (NaOCl). However, slight hemorrhage does not affect placement of MTA.

(Figure E) A mixture of MTA and water can now be placed into the prepared cavity against the pulpal wound and filling the entire cavity.

(Figure F) After setting (4–6 hours), a restoration can be placed to restore the tooth or bond the fractured crown fragment. While setting, the MTA serves as a temporary restoration. Thus, the patient should be instructed to avoid chewing or biting, as the material initially is quite soft.

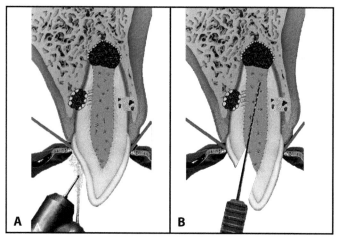

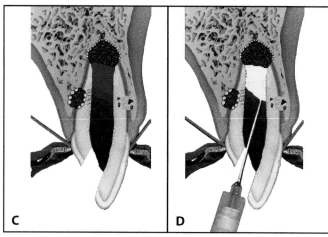

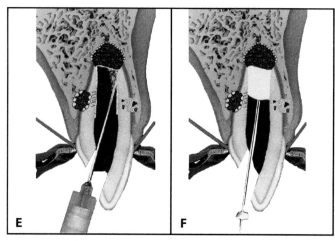

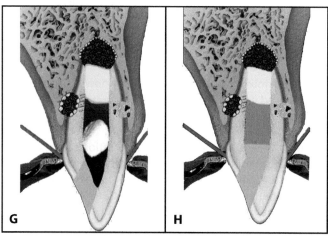

TREATMENT OF PULP NECROSIS IN IMMATURE TEETH

In situations where the pulp becomes necrotic before the root is fully developed, the apical opening is too large to create a stop for the root canal filling. Apexification procedures using calcium hydroxide have been performed with reasonable success.[189] The disadvantage in using calcium hydroxide for apexification is that it can take many months to obtain enough of an apical barrier to allow placement of a root canal filling.[188] Additionally, it now appears that long-term use can weaken dentin and result in cervical root fracture on slight impact or even with normal use.[191,192]

By using MTA as a physical barrier apically, a root canal filling can be placed immediately without waiting for a biological response.[193,194,201,202] Also, by minimizing exposure of root dentin to calcium hydroxide, there is less desiccation of dentin. The technique is as follows:

(Figure A) The tooth is isolated with a dental dam, the crown disinfected and an access cavity to the root canal prepared.

(Figure B) Extirpation of necrotic pulp tissue is done to a level apically where fresh bleeding from healthy tissue is encountered. This can be anywhere from several millimeters from the apex to flush with the apical foramen.

(Figure C) Root canal preparation in developing teeth requires a conservative approach, so as to preserve as much root dentin as possible. Hence minimal canal shaping is appropriate.

(Figure D) Disinfection of the root canal with sodium hypochlorite is followed by short-term (approximately 2–4 weeks) interim dressing with calcium hydroxide. The use of calcium hydroxide allows acceptable disinfection of the root canal system and provides a dry root canal, free of seepage of apical exudates. The coronal access opening must be sealed with a dependable temporary restoration.

(Figure E) At the next visit, the calcium hydroxide is removed and the canal is thoroughly irrigated with saline or sodium hypochlorite to obtain a debris-free canal.

(Figure F) Small increments of the MTA/water mixture are introduced into the canal and gently condensed. Length can be controlled using a rubber stopper on a plugger. No harm is done, however, with slight overfilling. When properly condensed, the apical MTA plug should be at least 4 mm thick. The entire canal can be filled with MTA (to the cervical level), or the coronal part of the canal can later be filled with gutta percha and sealer.

(Figure G) To allow setting, a moistened (water) cotton pellet is placed in the access cavity, which is then sealed with a temporary filling material. At the next visit the canal can be conventionally filled.

(Figure H) The temporary material and cotton pellet are removed and the apical plug is checked for setting hardness; it should not be vigorously probed, as the material can break. The canal is then irrigated, dried and filled, followed by a bonded coronal composite restoration.

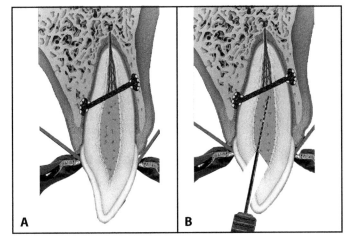

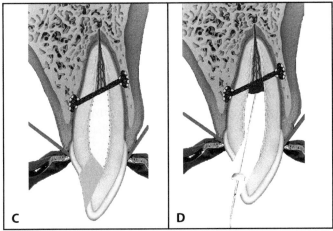

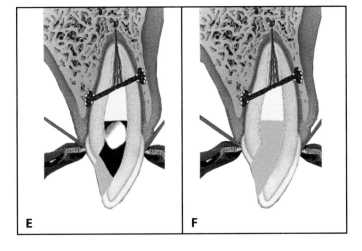

TREATMENT OF ROOT FRACTURES

(Figure A) In some instances, the coronal pulp undergoes necrosis, due to lack of revascularization, and the tooth requires root canal treatment to the fracture site in the root (see page 35).

(Figure B) The recommended procedure has been to isolate the tooth with a dental dam, extirpate the necrotic coronal pulp, and then clean and prepare the canal to the fracture site. This was then followed by placement of calcium hydroxide to obtain a hard tissue barrier at the level of fracture.[65] As in teeth with open apices, calcium hydroxide has been quite successful in inducing a hard tissue barrier but usually requires several months. Moreover, desiccation of dentin may also be a disadvantage in the use of calcium hydroxide.

(Figure C) In a manner similar to the open apex situation, calcium hydroxide is used for a short time (< 1 month) for disinfection purposes only. Instead of waiting for a hard tissue barrier to develop, MTA can be used to create a physical barrier at the fracture site. The technique is the same as described above for root canals with open apices, the only difference being the level of placement.

(Figure D) Small increments of the MTA/water mixture are introduced into the canal and gently condensed to the site of root fracture. As the distance from the fracture site to the coronal orifice may be quite short, it is advisable to fill the entire coronal root canal to the cervical level with MTA.

(Figure E) To allow setting, a moistened (water) cotton pellet is placed in the access cavity, which is then sealed with a temporary filling material.

(Figure F) At the next visit the access cavity can be restored with a bonded composite restoration to the level of the MTA after confirming that the MTA has set.

NOTES

_____
_____
_____
_____
_____
_____
_____
_____
_____

Decoronation of Ankylosed Teeth in Adolescents

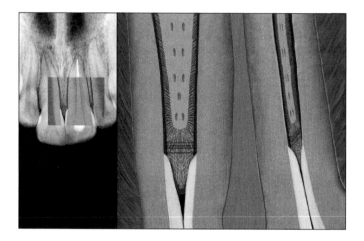

PERIODONTAL LIGAMENT PATHOLOGY AND ITS ROLE IN TOOTH ERUPTION

The eruption process during adolescence is dependent upon a normal and intact periodontal ligament. In cases of ankylosis normal eruption cannot take place, which creates a problem that can be severe in young patients, leading to progressive infraocclusion. This can also occur in adults where slow continuous eruption usually takes place.[207] The following periodontal ligament systems are essential for normal continuous eruption: an intact periodontal ligament structure (*Sharpey's fibers*), *cervical periosteal fibers* (green) that ensure alveolar vertical bone growth during the eruption process, and *interdental ligament fibers* (red) that maintain a slight interdental 'compressive' force between adjacent teeth.

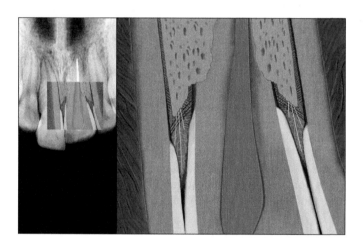

IMPORTANT MARGINAL PERIODONTAL STRUCTURES INVOLVED IN INFRAOCCLUSION

In case of pathosis involving the Sharpey's fiber structure (ankylosis), the following events take place: eruption is arrested and adjacent teeth are, via the interdental fibers, also slightly prevented from further eruption and are usually tilted towards the ankylosed tooth.[207]

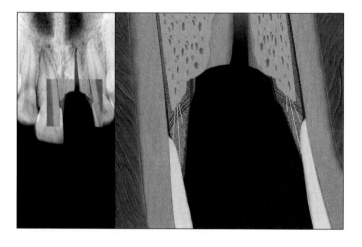

BIOLOGICAL CONSIDERATIONS IN DECORONATION

If the crown of the ankylosed tooth is removed, including disruption of the insertion of the interdental fibers and the cervical periosteal fibers, a number of healing events take place that will normalize the periodontal conditions.[207–210]

Traumatic Dental Injuries: A Manual, Third Edition   © J.O. Andreasen, L.K. Bakland, M.T. Flores, F.M. Andreasen and L. Andersson
Published 2011 by Blackwell Publishing Ltd

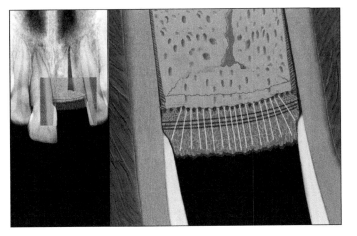

HEALING EVENTS AFTER DECORONATION

The fiber arrangement is normalized by uniting the interdental fibers and reforming new cervical periosteal fibers into the interdental bone, two events that allow the eruption process to continue. The decoronation procedure should include removal of 1 mm of the ankylosed root portion below the crest of the alveolar bone to prevent exposure of the root portion to the oral cavity.[207] Any root canal filling material present should be removed to allow the remaining ankylosed root portion to be replaced with bone during the ankylosis process.

When the anterior alveolar growth has been completed or the growth process has been very much reduced, the alveolar ridge will be at the optimal stage for reconstruction as the decoronated tooth has been able to maintain not only the labio-lingual bone width but also to allow continuous vertical growth of the alveolar process via the dento-periosteal fibers and development of a new periosteum in the decoronation area.

CLINICAL CASE OF DECORONATION

Decoronation performed on an ankylosed and infra-positioned central incisor in a 14-year-old boy (Figures A and B). Decoronation and removal of calcium hydroxyde from the root after root filling (Figures C and D). Temporary restoration (Figures E and F). Insertion of implant 10 years later (Figures G and H). Five-year follow-up (Figures I and J). Courtesy of B. Malmgren et al.[207] (2006).

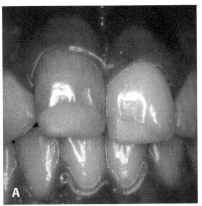
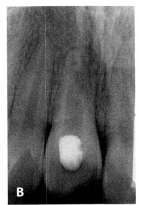
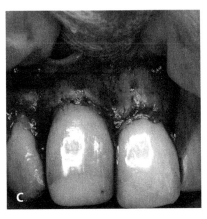
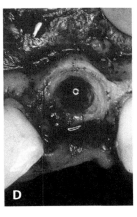
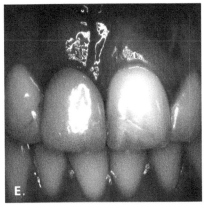
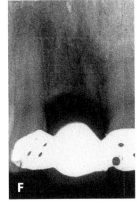
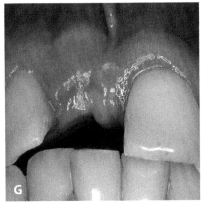
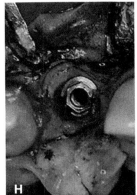
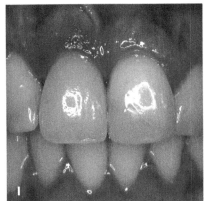
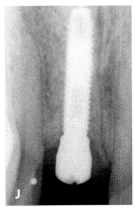

Predictors for Healing Complications

--- OBJECTIVES ---

1   Understand the relationship between healing complication predictors and the etiology of complications.

2   Recognize the relevance of healing complication predictors in treatment planning.

3   Recognize important predictors for pulp necrosis, root resorption, arrested root development, loss of marginal bone and tooth loss.

4   Recognize the use of predictors in an interactive program on www.dentaltraumaguide.org to assess the risk for individual trauma cases.

PULPAL HEALING AND PULPAL NECROSIS

Two main scenarios are involved in the development of infected pulp necrosis. The first is invasion of bacteria through dentinal tubules or directly to exposed pulpal tissue. The second follows rupture of the neurovascular supply to the pulp through the apical foramen, associated with a leak in the PDL, resulting in subsequent infection of the ischemic pulp.

The strongest healing predictor appears to be dislocation of the tooth in the socket (luxation diagnosis) followed by the size of the apical foramen.[211] The larger the diameter, the more likely the chances are for pulpal revascularization. Other predictors shown in the illustration have also been found to have implications.

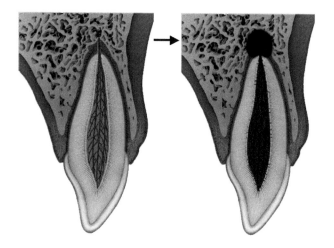

Predictors for pulp necrosis

- Size of apical foramen
- Luxation with displacement
- Length of pulp tissue (apex to coronal dentin)
- Compression of apical pulpal tissue (intrusion)
- Age
- External contaminants (avulsion)
- Dentin exposure
- Pulpal exposure
- Exactness of repositioning following displacement

PDL HEALING AND ROOT RESORPTION

A minor injury to the PDL, such as isolated rupture of PDL fibers, is generally followed by complete regeneration of the tissue. In more severe dental trauma (e.g. lateral luxation or intrusive luxation), in which tissue damage includes adjacent bony tissue, recruitment of osteoclasts often occurs, leading to resorption of the root surface. The result is *repair-related resorption* (surface resorption), *ankylosis-related resorption* or *infection-related resorption*.

PREDICTORS FOR ROOT RESORPTION

The most significant predictors appear to be the type and severity of the luxation injury (i.e. the extent of PDL damage and compression vs rupture of the PDL, see page 10).[211] Root resorption in avulsed/replanted teeth is very strongly related to extraoral dry time and choice of storage medium used before replantation. Other factors shown in the illustration have less association with the risk of root resorption.

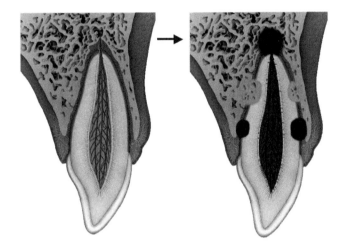

Predictors for root resorption

- Type of luxation
- Root development stage
- Compression of PDL
- Drying injury of PDL (avulsed teeth)
- Non-physiologic storage (avulsed teeth)
- Age
- Poorly performed root canal treatment
- Bacteria located in PDL, pulp or dentinal tubules

DISTURBED/ARRESTED ROOT DEVELOPMENT

Luxation injuries involving teeth with incomplete root development may cause damage to Hertwig's epithelial root sheath (HERS), a structure responsible for the morphology and shape of the root.[211] Any significant damage to this structure will result in partial or total arrest of further root formation through direct physical damage (e.g. intrusion or lateral luxation), or indirect damage related to delayed revascularization caused by incomplete repositioning. Among injuries leading to disturbances in root development are luxation with displacement, i.e. extrusion, lateral luxation, intrusion and avulsion with subsequent replantation and jaw fractures. Intrusion of primary teeth may also disturb root formation in permanent successors.

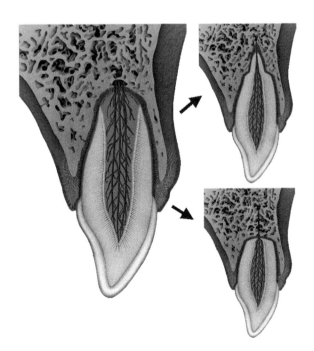

Predictors for disturbed root development

- Luxation with displacement
- Avulsion and replantation
- Inaccurate repositioning
- Alveolar fractures
- Intruded primary predecessors
- Jaw fractures

MARGINAL BONE HEALING AND BONE LOSS

The loss of marginal bone support following dental trauma is a rather rare occurrence which mainly affects teeth involved in intrusions, lateral luxations, jaw fractures and fractures of the alveolar process.[211] The etiology of marginal bone loss appears to be related to crushing of bone as well as exposure of the alveolar bone in severely displaced alveolar fractures. Teeth associated with alveolar fractures may suffer marginal breakdown, a finding that also applies to teeth associated with jaw fractures with marked displacement and late or unsuccessful repositioning. Loss of marginal bone is a rather frequent event after intrusion injuries and this factor becomes very prominent in the case of multiple adjacent intrusions. Lateral luxation injuries have a slight risk of initiating bone loss, especially orally.

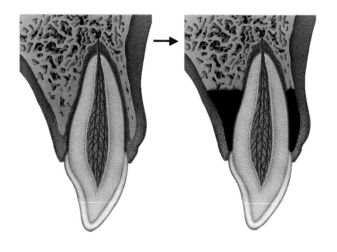

Predictors for marginal bone loss
- Compression of bone (intrusion, lateral luxation)
- Exposure of bone (alveolar and jaw fractures)
- Adjacent tooth/bone injury (multiple intrusions)
- Age

TOOTH SURVIVAL AND TOOTH LOSS

Tooth loss after trauma in the permanent dentition can be immediate or can occur later due to complications caused by insufficient pulpal or periodontal healing; and is primarily related to avulsion/replantation, intrusions, root fractures and crown-root fractures.[211]

Avulsion injuries have generally a poor prognosis due to the deleterious effect of extraoral time and storage upon the PDL and the pulp, damage which leads to progressive root resorption. In *intrusive luxations*, owing to compression of the PDL and the pulp, numerous healing complications can occur. These include a high frequency of progressive root resorption, pulp necrosis and loss of marginal bone. Despite this, a significant number of teeth still survive for long periods of time.

Root fractures (intra-alveolar) represent a complex injury. In approximately 25% of root fractures, pulp necrosis occurs. These teeth have been found to respond very well to endodontic treatment, but tooth loss may occur later due to loss of bone support. This also applies to root fractures located in the cervical one-third of the root where tooth loss may occur for the same reason.

Teeth with *crown-root fractures* have traditionally been considered hopeless to preserve and are often extracted at the time of injury. There are, however, a number of procedures that should be considered before removing the damaged tooth (see page 33).

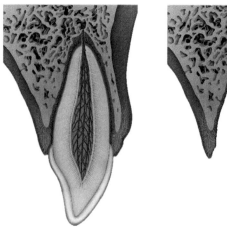
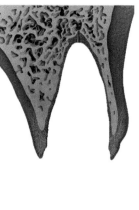

Predictors for tooth loss
- Avulsed teeth where replantation is not indicated
- Complications following replantation of avulsed teeth
- Intrusion with complications
- Crown-root fractures
- Root fractures, cervical

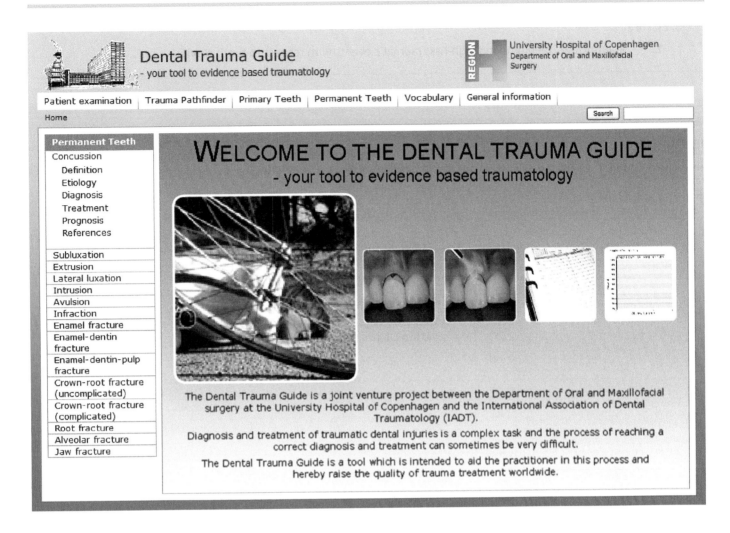

USE OF PREDICTORS IN AN INTERACTIVE DENTAL TRAUMA GUIDE

At the Trauma Center in Copenhagen, a series of long-term follow-up studies covering all types of injuries affecting primary and permanent dentitions have been performed since 1970.[212] Data from these studies have now been combined into a common database containing nine fracture and six luxation types and combinations of these, resulting in close to 50 trauma entities being fully covered for both the permanent and primary dentitions. The database has now been placed on the internet (www.dentaltraumaguide.org).[213]

PROGNOSIS ESTIMATION FOR INDIVIDUAL PATIENTS

A program has been developed in which a patient's specific data can be fed into the database.[213] Based on the information supplied, the database can provide the survival statistics for pulpal and periodontal healing, loss of marginal bone and tooth survival for the specific injury. This is achieved by matching the actual injury and predictors to a subsection of the database with a similar injury type and similar predictors.

NOTES

_____

_____

_____

_____

_____

_____

_____

_____

_____

_____

_____

Tooth Survival in the Permanent Dentition

┌─ OBJECTIVE ───┐
│ **1**   Identify low-, medium- and high-risk traumatic events with respect to tooth survival. │
└───┘

DESCRIPTION

The following graphs represent one study on the long-term prognosis of various trauma entities.[214–224] Based on the findings, prognosis for each trauma entity is identified as *good*, *fair* or *poor*.

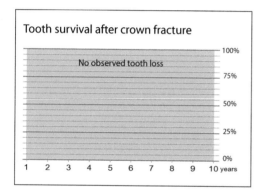

CROWN FRACTURES

Irrespective of presence or absence of pulp exposure, crown fractures have a *good* long-term prognosis.[214–218]

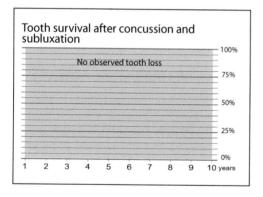

CONCUSSION AND SUBLUXATION

Both trauma entities have *good* long-term tooth survival.[214–218]

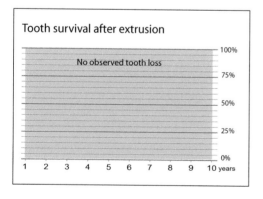

EXTRUSION

Tooth survival is to a certain degree related to tooth development at time of injury. The chance of long-term survival is *good*.[214–218]

Traumatic Dental Injuries: A Manual, Third Edition   © J.O. Andreasen, L.K. Bakland, M.T. Flores, F.M. Andreasen and L. Andersson
Published 2011 by Blackwell Publishing Ltd

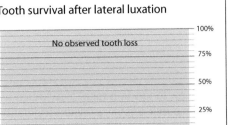

Tooth survival after lateral luxation

LATERAL LUXATION

Tooth survival is to a certain degree related to tooth development at time of injury. The chance of long-term survival is *good*.[214]

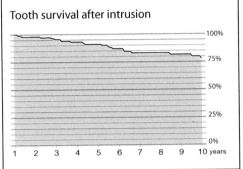

Tooth survival after intrusion

INTRUSION

Tooth survival is strongly related to tooth development at time of injury. The leading cause of failure is progression of infection-related and/or ankylosis-related resorption. Due to generally *fair* long-term survival, treatment alternatives (e.g. orthodontic space closure, transplantation of premolars, implants or fixed prosthetics) may be considered, especially if ankylosis-related (replacement) resorption occurs.[220, 221]

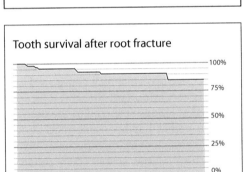

Tooth survival after root fracture

ROOT FRACTURES

Long-term survival is strongly related to the type of healing. This graph illustrates that both healing with hard tissue (HT), connective tissue (CT) and successfully treated pulp necrosis (GT) have *fair* long-term prognoses.[222] The root fractures with the greatest risk of tooth loss appear to be the ones located in the cervical one-third of the root.[222]

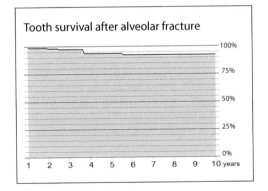

Tooth survival after alveolar fracture

ALVEOLAR FRACTURE

There is a good long-term survival with longer observation periods.[224]

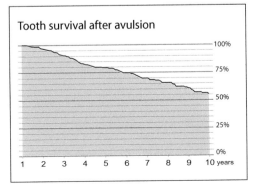

Tooth survival after avulsion

AVULSION AND REPLANTATION

The most significant factors determining long-term survival appear to be storage time and storage media.[223] Due to the many variations in the combination of these two factors, it is not possible in this context to present survival scenarios for all possible combinations. In a large long-term clinical study of 400 replanted teeth, a *fair* survival was found.[223]

Information for the Patient About Dental Trauma

┌─ OBJECTIVE ───┐
│   │
│   **1**   Provide information for patients who have suffered a traumatic dental injury.   │
│   │
└───┘

When teeth or jaws have been injured, many questions arise. Can the injury be treated? How long will it take? How much will it cost? What is the prognosis for traumatized teeth? Is treatment covered by insurance or public agencies? When the dentist is faced with an emergency, it is of utmost importance to give emotional support to the patient as well as to the stressed and anxious parents. An attempt will be made to answer such questions here.[225-228] The following material can be copied and used as handouts for patients.

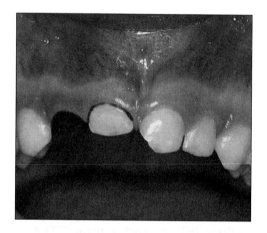

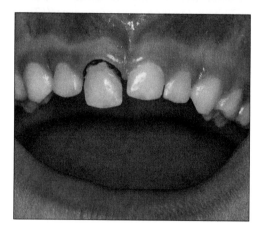

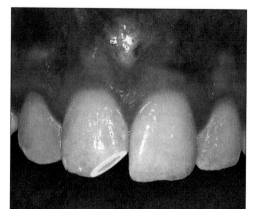

PRIMARY (MILK) TOOTH INJURIES

Often there is just loosening of the primary (milk) tooth. Inform the parents to wait for the loosened primary tooth to tighten up, which usually happens within a few weeks. In this healing period, it is very important that the child avoids hard foods, but that doesn't mean a liquid diet.

In some cases, the tooth is forced into the jaw. An X-ray will be taken to determine the extent of injury and to discover whether the permanent tooth bud – which lies just under the primary tooth root – has also been affected. If this is the case, it may be necessary to remove the primary tooth to improve the chance of normal development of the permanent tooth. If the primary tooth is not too close to the permanent tooth germ the displaced primary tooth may grow out again within 2–4 months.

In rare cases, an infection of the root can develop, which will cause swelling and redness around the injured tooth. It is very important that this infection be treated by the dentist immediately, so that it doesn't spread to the permanent tooth. Record in the chart that the parent has been informed about possible complications in the developing permanent teeth, especially following intrusion, avulsion and alveolar fracture injuries sustained in children under 3 years of age.[228]

FRACTURE OF PERMANENT TEETH

Fractures of the crown of the tooth can vary in extent. If only a corner of the enamel is involved, usually only slight grinding is necessary.

If the fracture has exposed dentin, it is necessary to restore the tooth either with a tooth-colored material or by bonding the original fragment. If the broken tooth fragment is available, it can be reattached with a special glue. This can be done at the time of injury or at a later date; but it is important that the fragment be kept moist, by storing it in a glass of water, and brought to the dentist.

If the nerve is exposed, it must be covered with a special material to help the nerve heal. This usually takes 2–3 months. However, the final restoration can be made over this dressing in the form of either tooth-colored material or reattachment of the tooth fragment. Porcelain veneers or crowns can be made later, once the child has grown up.

Traumatic Dental Injuries: A Manual, Third Edition   © J.O. Andreasen, L.K. Bakland, M.T. Flores, F.M. Andreasen and L. Andersson
Published 2011 by Blackwell Publishing Ltd

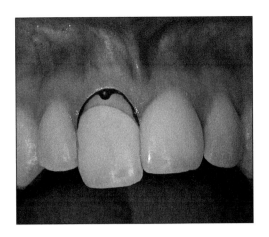

LOOSENED OR DISPLACED PERMANENT TEETH

The tooth should be put back in place in the jaw and a splint applied to protect the loosened tooth in the healing period. The splint will usually be removed after 1–4 weeks, depending on the type of injury. Chewing is permitted, but hard foods should be avoided. If the splint becomes loose, it should be re-bonded. During the healing period, when traumatized teeth are splinted, the patient should avoid contact sports.

In some cases loosening of the tooth means that the nerve dies. The dead nerve must be removed and replaced by a root filling (root canal filling). In rare cases this can lead to discoloration of the crown of the tooth. Tooth bleaching or a porcelain crown can correct this problem in older patients.

FRACTURE OF THE JAW

In these cases it is often necessary to place splints on the teeth in the upper and lower jaw and then bind the lower jaw to the upper. This is done to ensure that the fracture heals in the right position. Normally the jaws must be bound together for 3–6 weeks, depending on the fracture's severity. A special liquid diet is prescribed during this period.

DIET

In some cases, when the teeth have been loosened, a splint will not be applied. Instead, a soft diet will be prescribed for the first 14 days, to protect the injured teeth. A soft diet means no hard foods, but not necessarily a liquid diet.

ORAL HYGIENE

Meticulous cleansing of the teeth and gums is necessary for rapid healing and it should start as soon as possible after injury. Daily oral hygiene includes the following:
- Rinse your mouth thoroughly with one tablespoon of chlorhexidine twice a day for one week. For children under 7 years, topical use of chlorhexidine is indicated.
- Careful tooth brushing after every meal, with a soft toothbrush, working from the gums to the teeth in the upper and lower jaws.
- After tooth brushing, make sure that splints and teeth are completely clean.
- If there are associated lip injuries, use of lip balm during the healing period will avoid dryness.

FOLLOW-UP EXAMINATION

In some cases, it is necessary to take X-rays 2, 4, 6 or 8 weeks and 1 year after injury to control healing. X-rays are taken to discover possible late healing complications, such as infection of the root or jaw.

PROGNOSIS OF TREATMENT

When treatment has been carried out, the patient and/or parents must receive information about prognosis for the injured teeth.

INJURY REPORT

A written report including cause, type of injury, treatment and prognosis must be completed for school-related accidents and occupational injuries. Also, this report will be useful for a court trial when dental injuries are a result of violence, assaults or traffic accidents.

INSURANCE

Consult your dentist with regard to collection of the needed information for insurance purposes. The dentist should have a general knowledge about dental insurance coverage following accidents.

Information for the Public About Dental Trauma

OBJECTIVES

1 Inform the community about the importance of preventing and treating dental trauma.

2 Describe specific ways, suitable for different age groups, in which dental trauma can be prevented.

3 Recommend appropriate emergency measures to be taken immediately following dental trauma.

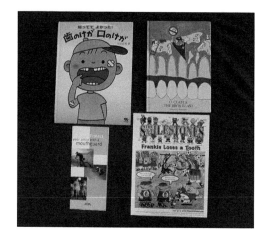

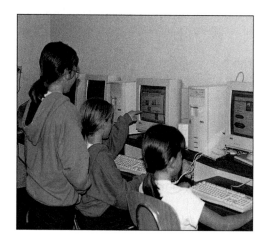

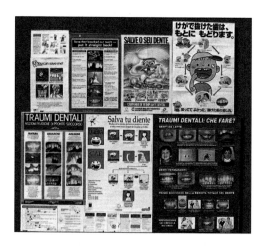

DEVELOPING PUBLIC DENTAL TRAUMA AWARENESS

Parents and preschool teachers should receive guidance in injury prevention and associated risks following traumatic oral-dental injuries sustained by young children.[229–231] Emotional and esthetic long-term consequences may be emphasized to create awareness in order to avoid intentional and non-intentional injuries.[232] The dentist should give advice to school-age children and athletes on the type and proper use of mouthguards in contact sports such as rugby, hockey, football, volleyball and basketball.[233–235] Because amateur players are more at risk than professionals, injury prevention campaigns addressing the need for protective devices in sports and bicycling can increase awareness and use. This can be achieved through legislation or regulation.

Education in the management of acute dental injuries focusing on tooth avulsion has had growing interest among those in the dental profession.[236–241] However, the psychological, emotional and economic consequences of such injuries have not had high priority in public health campaigns. The proposed campaign must be focused so as to present its message clearly, making the population aware of its role in saving teeth at the site of accident or as a result of violence.[242,243] To reach this goal, dental school curricula and the dental profession should be updated with the IADT current Guidelines for the Management of Traumatic Dental Injuries.[244] By attending continuing education courses on dental trauma, dentists become more conscious of their role and commitment to educate school teachers, parents, health care personnel and the general public. It would seem that public education needs a more comprehensive analysis.[245,246] Collaboration of behavioral science-related professionals could be considered in order to support and reassure emergency health care personnel and the lay public in their willingness to replant an avulsed permanent tooth.

INTERNET USE IN TRAUMA EDUCATION AND PREVENTION

The Internet is a useful communication tool. It is an effective form of spreading knowledge, accessible at very low cost to many potential users. An educational cartoon video promoting the use of mouthguards is strongly recommended for injury prevention programs for children.[248] Information for the public can be found at professional organizations such as IADT, AAPD, IAPD, AAE and on government and university websites. Also, PubMed is a valuable database of scientific information where dentists and lay people can also search for dental trauma knowledge.[247] Recently, an interactive *Dental Trauma Guide* has been developed,[248] with illustrations and animations to improve knowledge about dental traumatology worldwide and thereby improve the quality of treatment. The *Dental Trauma Guide* has been sponsored by the *International Association of Dental Traumatology* (IADT), dental companies and dental organizations (AAE and EAPD). The *Dental Trauma Guide* is available at www.dentaltraumaguide.org

Traumatic Dental Injuries: A Manual, Third Edition   © J.O. Andreasen, L.K. Bakland, M.T. Flores, F.M. Andreasen and L. Andersson
Published 2011 by Blackwell Publishing Ltd

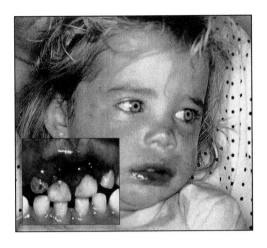

TRAUMA BROCHURES AND POSTERS

Recent studies have shown the effectiveness of educational material in the form of brochures and posters[236,238] associated with a lecture in improving the knowledge of the treatment of tooth avulsion by school teachers and parents.[237-239] Furthermore, the *International Association of Dental Traumatology* has developed the 'Save a Tooth' poster directed at the public for the emergency management of the avulsed permanent tooth at the site of the injury. It has been translated into Spanish, Portuguese, French, Icelandic, Italian, and recently into Arabic and Catalonian. The illustrations were created by designers from the University of Valparaiso, Chile. The poster, in several languages, is available at the IADT website: www.iadt-dentaltrauma.org

FIRST-AID AND TREATMENT OF TRAUMA TO PRIMARY TEETH

Recommendations to the public when responding to dental trauma in young children should include the following measures:

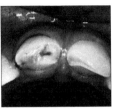
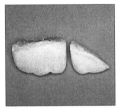

- Wash the wound with plenty of running water. Generally, dental trauma includes injuries to the adjacent soft tissue.
- Stop bleeding by compressing the injured area with gauze or cotton wool for 5 minutes.
- Seek emergency treatment from a pediatric dentist, an oral and maxillofacial surgeon, a general dentist or an emergency clinic.
- Important: it is not recommended to replant avulsed primary teeth.

FIRST-AID AND TREATMENT OF TRAUMA TO PERMANENT TEETH

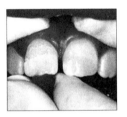
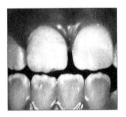

Tooth fractures (broken teeth), luxations (loosened or displaced teeth) and avulsions (complete loss of the tooth) are the most frequent injuries to the permanent teeth which could have an improved outcome if the public is well informed about appropriate first-aid measures.

FIRST-AID FOR A CROWN FRACTURE

With a crown fracture, the broken piece of tooth may be repositioned using dental adhesives and composite resins.
- Find the tooth fragment and place it in a glass of water.
- Seek dental treatment immediately.

FIRST-AID FOR AN AVULSED *PERMANENT* TOOTH

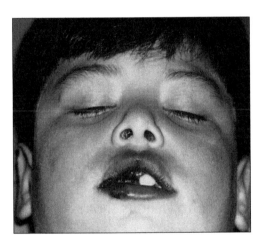

Often a permanent tooth can be saved through appropriate first-aid and immediate treatment.

- Find the tooth and pick it up by the crown.
- If the tooth is dirty, wash briefly (10 seconds) under cold running water and put it back into the tooth socket.
- The patient should be instructed to keep the tooth in position by gently pressing a gauze or handkerchief. If this is not possible, place the tooth in a glass of milk. The tooth can also be transported in the mouth, keeping it between the teeth and the cheek. *Avoid storage in water*.
- Seek emergency dental treatment immediately.

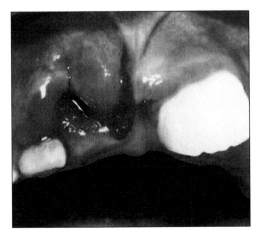

Important: when providing first-aid information for tooth avulsion, be aware that the public recognizes basic knowledge of the tooth. An illustration of the crown and root (a real picture preferably), and the way to put the tooth back – with the labial side of the crown facing front – is of utmost importance.

Prevention of Traumatic Dental Injuries

OBJECTIVES

1   Identify medium- and high-risk sports.
2   Describe preventive measures.
3   Describe effects of prevention measures.

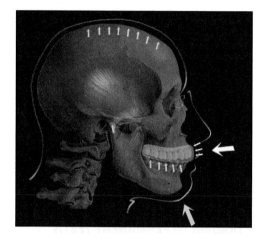

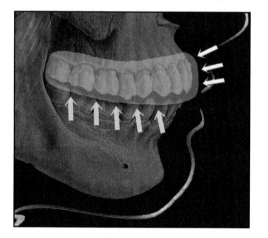

MECHANISM OF MOUTHGUARD PROTECTION

All sports activities are connected with a certain risk of orofacial injuries from falls, collisions and contact with hard surfaces. Contact sports, such as ice hockey, football, handball, soccer and basketball, with their high risk of collisions at high speed, are especially prone to result in dental and other injuries.[249-260] Clinical and experimental evidence suggests that mouthguards can help to distribute energy from impact, and thereby reduce the risk of severe injury.[255-265]

The mechanism of mouthguard protection varies according to the energy and direction of impact. If the impact hits the base of the mandible, the cushioning effect of the elastic mouthguard between the mandible and the maxilla reduces the force of impact occlusally, as well as preventing crown and crown-root fractures. In the condylar region, the forces of impact are also reduced. With a frontal impact, the impact force is reduced again due to the material's elasticity and by distribution of forces over a greater area.[261-265] Whether this implies that the risk of fracture is replaced by risk of tooth luxations remains to be examined. In several types of sports the use of mouthguards seems to reduce the risk of dental injuries.[259]

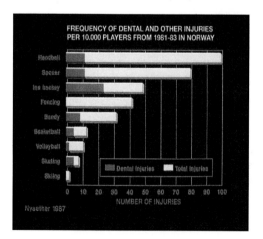

FREQUENCY OF DENTAL AND OTHER INJURIES
PER 10.000 PLAYERS FROM 1981-83 IN NORWAY

Nysether 1987

DENTAL AND OTHER INJURIES RELATED TO VARIOUS SPORTS

Based on insurance records from Norway, a very precise documentation of dental and other injuries exists.[266] In this report, ice hockey was found to be associated with the highest risks followed by handball and soccer.[266] Sports-related injuries are usually very costly.[267]

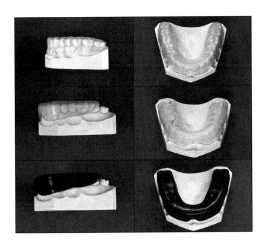

VARIOUS TYPES OF MOUTH PROTECTORS

Stock (or unfitted) mouthguards are of latex rubber or polyvinyl chloride, usually made in three sizes and promoted to be universally fitting, the advantage being their low cost. However, they have been found to impede both speech and breathing, as they can only be kept in place by occlusion. There is no evidence that they can redistribute forces of impact.

Mouth-formed (boil and bite) mouthguards are fitted from a manufactured kit consisting of a fairly rigid outer shell and a soft resilient heat-cured or self-cured lining. These protectors have the advantage of a better fit and low cost. A recent study has shown less severe orodental injuries when boil and bite mouthguards were distributed free of charge to young adult amateur sportsmen.[268] However, free distribution is not enough for amateur players to become aware of the use of mouthguards unless they are properly motivated and educated on prevention of dental injuries.[268]

Custom-made mouthguards are individually processed by a dentist or dental technician on plaster models of the athlete's dental arches. The pressure-laminated variety seems to afford the best protection.[261,269] These protectors, while significantly more expensive than stock or mouth-formed mouthguards, have been found to be acceptable and comfortable by many athletes.

FACE MASKS

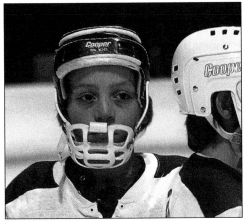

Face masks are used extensively in ice hockey. Since the use of helmets, face-masks and mouthguards became mandatory in organized contact sports, such as football and ice hockey in the USA and many other countries, they have been found to be very effective in protecting players from orofacial injuries.[270] In a study of ice hockey players, it was shown that both full and partial facial protection reduce injuries to the eyes and face from 159 to 23 injuries per 1000 player–game hours.[250]

EFFECT OF MOUTHGUARDS AND FACE MASK PROTECTION IN AMERICAN FOOTBALL

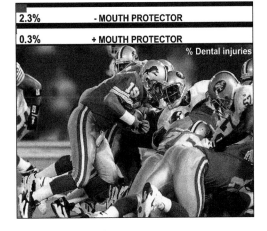

2.3% - MOUTH PROTECTOR
0.3% + MOUTH PROTECTOR
% Dental injuries

Roberts[271] studied the incidence of dental injuries in American football over a period of 14 years in Wisconsin, USA. During this period, a dramatic reduction in the annual incidence was seen – first with the introduction of face masks and later by the addition of mouthguards. Similar figures have been reported in Finland.[272]

EFFECT OF MOUTHGUARD PROTECTION IN ICE HOCKEY

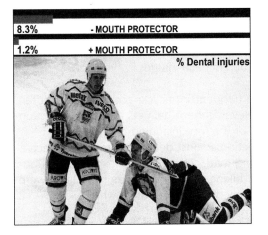

8.3% - MOUTH PROTECTOR
1.2% + MOUTH PROTECTOR
% Dental injuries

Ice hockey is the contact sport that is associated with the greatest risk of orofacial injury.[273] A study of professional Canadian hockey players showed that 62% had lost one or more incisors.[255] The use of mouthguards in ice hockey in Canada has been shown to decrease the annual rate of dental injuries from 8.3% to 1.2%.[255]

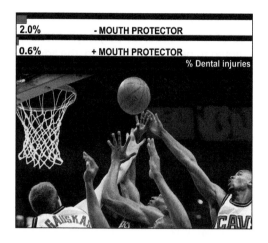

2.0%	- MOUTH PROTECTOR
0.6%	+ MOUTH PROTECTOR
	% Dental injuries

EFFECT OF MOUTHGUARD PROTECTION IN BASKETBALL

An American study reported a dramatic decrease in the frequency of orofacial injuries in players using mouthguards in the 1986–1987 varsity basketball season.[274] About two-thirds of the injuries recorded consisted of lacerations and bruises. A recent prospective study led to the conclusion that custom-fitted mouthguards did not significantly affect rates of brain concussions or oral soft tissue injuries, but could significantly reduce the morbidity and expense resulting from dental injuries in men's college basketball.[275]

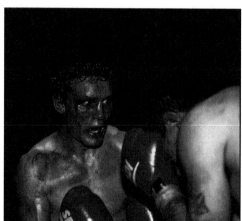

EFFECT OF MOUTHGUARDS IN BOXING

Boxing was the first sports activity where the need for mouthguards was recognized. In the boxing world championship held in Cuba in 1975, no oral injuries were found after examination of 250 boxers, all of them wearing mouthguards.[259,276]

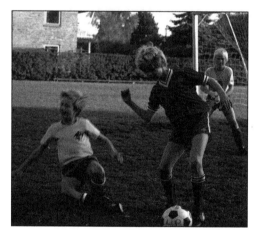

EFFECT OF MOUTHGUARDS IN SOCCER

Soccer is probably the most widespread sports activity in the world today. Being a contact sport, it is known to involve a high risk of injuries especially to extremities, but also oral injuries are frequent. This risk is especially high for goal keepers and forwards and is also strongly related to the more experienced teams.[266]

Studies from the USA and Japan reported oral injury incidences of 28% and 32%, respectively, among high school soccer players in a 2-year season.[253,254] In both studies, almost none of the players used mouthguards.

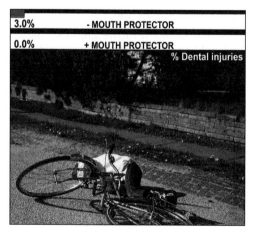

3.0%	- MOUTH PROTECTOR
0.0%	+ MOUTH PROTECTOR
	% Dental injuries

EFFECT OF HELMET PROTECTION IN BICYCLING

Head injuries are very frequent in bicycle accidents. In Victoria, Australia, mandatory helmet protection was introduced in 1990. After 1 year of helmet legislation, there was a 48% reduction in head injuries.[277]

Oral and maxillofacial injuries are frequent in bicycle accidents in children aged younger than 15 years. However, current helmets offer no protection against injuries to the lower part of the face including dental injuries,[278–280] whereas mouthguards offer protection against dental injuries.[265] In a recent study from Switzerland it was found that 5.7% of athletes experienced traumatic dental injuries in mountain biking.[281] Even when most athletes were aware about mouthguards, only a few of them used them while biking.[281]

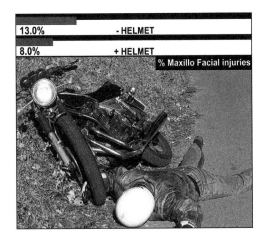

EFFECT OF HELMET PROTECTION IN MOTORCYCLE-RELATED INJURIES

Motorcycle injuries are a major source of fatal and nonfatal head trauma in the USA. The use of helmets reduces maxillofacial injuries by up to 50%.[282,283]

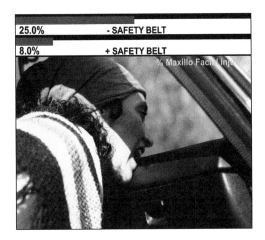

EFFECT OF SAFETY BELTS IN MOTOR VEHICLE-RELATED INJURIES

Motor vehicle-related injuries are known to lead to frequent dental and maxillofacial injuries. Front-seat passengers are particularly at risk, due to collision with the front panel or steering wheel. In a study from the USA, it was shown that the use of safety belts reduced the frequency of facial injuries from 25% to 8%.[284]

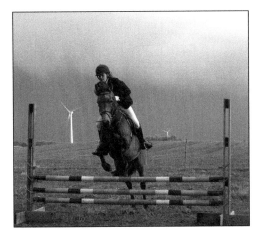

EFFECT OF HELMET PROTECTION IN HORSEBACK RIDING

Horseback riding is known not only to be a sporting activity with a very high incidence of injury, but also of severe injuries, sometimes with a fatal outcome. These injuries are usually caused by falls from the horse, collision with branches when riding in forests or by horse kicks when standing behind the horse. The use of helmets, especially with a strap protecting the chin, can prevent some of these injuries. However, no statistics exist on the extent of prevention.

NOTES

Appendix 1

Emergency record for acute dental trauma

Patient's name	
Birth date	

Date of examination:	Referred by:
Time of examination:	Referring diagnosis:

General medical history: any serious illness? ☐ yes ☐ no
If yes, explain.
Any allergy? ☐ yes ☐ no
If yes, explain.
Have you been vaccinated against tetanus? ☐ yes ☐ no
If yes, when.

Previous dental injuries: ☐ yes ☐ no
If yes,
   When?
   Which teeth were injured?
   Treatment given and by whom?

Present dental injury:
   Date: Time:
   Where?
   How?

Have you had or have now *headache?* ☐ yes ☐ no

Have you had or have now *nausea?* ☐ yes ☐ no

Have you had or have now *vomiting?* ☐ yes ☐ no

Were you *unconscious* at the time of injury? ☐ yes ☐ no
If yes, for how long (minutes)?
Can you *remember* what happened before, ☐ yes ☐ no
during or after the accident?

Is there pain from *cold air?* ☐ yes ☐ no
If yes, *which teeth?*

Is there pain or tenderness from *occlusion?* ☐ yes ☐ no
If yes, *which teeth?*

Constant pain? ☐ yes ☐ no
If yes, *which teeth?*

Treatment elsewhere? ☐ yes ☐ no
If yes, *what treatment?*

Traumatic Dental Injuries: A Manual, Third Edition © J.O. Andreasen, L.K. Bakland, M.T. Flores, F.M. Andreasen and L. Andersson
Published 2011 by Blackwell Publishing Ltd

Emergency record for acute dental trauma

page 2

After *avulsion,* the following information is needed:
Where were the teeth found (dirt, asphalt, floor, etc.)?
When were the teeth found?
Were the teeth *dirty?*
How were the teeth *stored?*
Were the teeth *rinsed* and *with what* prior to replantation?
When were the teeth replanted?
Was *tetanus antitoxoid* given?
Were *antibiotics* given?
Antibiotic?
Dosage?

Objective examination

Is the patient's general condition affected?	yes	no
If yes, *pulse*		
blood pressure		
pupillary reflex		
cerebral condition		
Objective findings beyond the head and neck?	yes	no
If yes, *type* and *location*		
Objective findings within the head and neck?	yes	no
If yes, *type* and *location*		

Objective examination – Extraoral findings (contd.)

Bleeding from nose, or rhinitis	yes	no
Bleeding from ext. auditory canal	yes	no
Double vision or limited eye movement	yes	no
Palpable signs of fracture of facial skeleton	yes	no
If yes, *location of fracture*		

Objective examination – Intraoral findings

Lesions of the *oral mucosa*	yes	no
If yes, *type* and *location*		
Gingival lesion	yes	no
If yes, *type* and *location*		
Tooth fracture	yes	no
If yes, *type* and *location*		
Alveolar fracture	yes	no
If yes, *type* and *location*		

Supplemental information:

General condition of the dentition

Caries	poor	fair	good
Periodontal status	poor	fair	good
Horizontal occlusal relationship	undr bite	over jet	norm
Vertical occlusal relationship	deep	open	norm

Emergency record for acute dental trauma

Radiographic findings
Tooth dislocation
Root fracture
Bone fracture
Pulp canal obliteration
Root resorption

Photographic registration   [yes]   [no]

Diagnoses (check appropriate boxes and designate tooth no. or indicate correct anatomical region)

□ Infraction   □ Skin abrasion
□ Enamel fracture   □ Skin laceration
□ Enamel-dentine fracture   □ Skin contusion
□ Enamel-dentine pulp fracture

□ Crown-root fracture without pulp exposure   □ Mucosal abrasion
□ Crown-root fracture with pulp exposure   □ Mucosal laceration
                   □ Mucosal contusion

□ Root fracture
□ Alveolar fracture   □ Gingival abrasion
□ Mandibular fracture   □ Gingival laceration
□ Maxillary fracture   □ Gingival contusion

□ Concussion
□ Subluxation   *Supplementary remarks:*
□ Extrusion
□ Lateral luxation
□ Intrusion
□ Avulsion

Treatment plan
At time of injury: *Final therapy:*
Repositioning (time finished)
Fixation (time finished)
Pulpal therapy (time finished)
Dentinal coverage (time finished)

Chart re-read by examining dentist   [yes]   [no]

Appendix 2

Clinical examination form for the time of injury and follow-up examinations

		Tooth no.	12		11		21		22	
T I M E		Date								

		Tooth color
		  normal
		  yellow
		  red
		  grey
		  crown restoration								

O F		Displacement (mm)
		  intruded
		  extruded
		  protruded
		  retruded								

I N J U R Y		Loosening (0-3)								
		Tenderness to percussion (+/−)								
		Pulp test (value)								
		Ankylosis tone (+/−)								
		Occlusal contact (+/−)								
C O N T R O L		Fistula (+/−)								
		Gingivitis (+/−)								
		Gingival retraction (mm)								
		Abnormal pocketing (+/−)								

Each column represents an examination of a given tooth. The first column for each tooth gives the values from the time of injury. *Only* the parameters listed in the top half of the form ("Time of injury") are to be recorded at the time of injury. The information from this examination as well as the information collected on the emergency record are used to determine the final diagnoses for the injured teeth. Those parameters *and* the last four (fistula, gingivitis, gingival retraction, abnormal pocketing) are to be registered at all follow-up controls.

Appendix 3

Clinical and radiographic findings with the various luxation types

Findings	Concussion	Subluxation	Extrusion	Lateral Luxation	Intrusion
Clinical					
Abnormal mobility	−	+	+	−(+)	−(+)
Tenderness to percussion	+	+(−)*	+/−	−(+)	−(+)
Percussion sound**	normal	dull	dull	metallic	metallic
Response to pulp testing	+/−	+/−	−(+)	−(+)	−(+)
Clinical dislocation	−	−	+	+	+
Radiographic dislocation	−	−	+	+	+

* A sign in parentheses indicates a finding of rare occurrence.
** Teeth with incomplete root formation and teeth with marginal or periapical inflammatory lesions will also elicit a dull percussion sound.

References

EPIDEMIOLOGY OF TRAUMATIC DENTAL INJURIES

1. **Glendor U, Marcenes W, Andreasen JO**. Classification, epidemiology and etiology. In: Andreasen JO, Andreasen FM, Andersson L, (eds), *Textbook and Color Atlas of Traumatic Injuries to the Teeth* (4th edn). Oxford: Blackwell, 2007. pp. 217–254.
2. **Glendor U, Halling A, Andersson L, Eilert-Petersson E**. Incidence of traumatic tooth injuries in children and adolescents in country of Västmanland Sweden. *Swed Dent J* 1996;20:15–28.
3. **Crona-Larson G, Noren JG**. Luxation injuries to permanent teeth – a retrospective study of aetiological factors. *Endod Dent Traumatol* 1985;5:176–179.
4. **Petersson EE, Andersson L, Sörensen S**. Traumatic oral vs non-oral injuries. *Swed Dent J* 1997;21:55–86.

PATHOPHYSIOLOGY AND CONSEQUENCES OF DENTAL TRAUMA

5. **Gottrup F, Storgård Jensen S, Andreasen JO**. Wound healing subsequent to injury. In: Andreasen JO, Andreasen FM, Andersson L (eds), *Textbook and Color Atlas of Traumatic Injuries to the Teeth* (4th edn). Oxford: Blackwell, 2007. pp. 1–61.
6. **Andreasen JO, Løvschall H**. Response of oral tissues to trauma. In: Andreasen JO, Andreasen FM, Andersson L (eds), *Textbook and Color Atlas of Traumatic Injuries to the Teeth* (4th edn). Oxford: Blackwell, 2007. pp. 62–113.
7. **Andreasen JO**. Experimental dental traumatology: development of a model for external root resorption. *Endod Dent Traumatol* 1987;3:269–287.
8. **Andreasen JO**. Review of root resorption systems and models. Etiology of root resorption and the homeostatic mechanisms of the periodontal ligament. In: Davidovitch Z (ed.), *The Biological Mechanisms of Tooth Eruption and Root Resorption*. Birmingham: EBSCO Media, 1988. pp. 9–21.
9. **Andreasen JO, Andreasen FM, Mèjare I, Cvek M**. Healing of 400 intra-alveolar root fractures. 2. Effect of treatment factors such as treatment delay, repositioning, splinting type, period and antibiotics. *Dent Traumatol* 2004;20:203–211.
10. **Andreasen JO**. The effect of splinting upon periodontal healing after replantation of permanent incisors in monkeys. *Acta Odont Scand* 1975;33:313–323.
11. **Cvek M, Cleaton-Jones P, Austin J, Kling M, Lownie J, Fatti P**. Effect of topical application of doxycycline on pulp revascularization and periodontal healing in reimplanted monkey incisors. *Endod Dent Traumatol* 1990;6:170–176.
12. **Cvek M, Cleaton-Jones P, Austin J, King M, Lownie J, Fatti P**. Pulp revascularization in reimplanted immature monkey incisors – predictability and the effect of antibiotic systemic prophylaxis. *Endod Dent Traumatol* 1990;6:157–169.
13. **Hammarström L, Blomlöf L, Feiglin B, Andersson L, Lindskog S**. Replantation of teeth and antibiotic treatment. *Endod Dent Traumatol* 1986;2:51–57.
14. **Sae-Lim V, Wang CY, Choi GW, Trope M**. The effect of systemic tetracycline on resorption of dried replanted dogs' teeth. *Endod Dent Traumatol* 1998;14:127–132.
15. **Andreasen JO, Jensen SS, Sae-Lim V**. The role of antibiotics in preventing healing complications after traumatic dental injuries: a literature review. *Endod Topics* 2006;14:80–92.
16. **Yanpiset K, Trope M**. Pulp revascularization of replanted immature dog teeth after different treatment methods. *Endod Dent Traumatol* 2000;16:211–217.

CLASSIFICATION OF DENTAL INJURIES

17. **Andreasen JO, Andreasen FM**. Classification, etiology and epidemiology of traumatic dental injuries. In: Andreasen JO, Andreasen FM (eds), Textbook and Color Atlas of Traumatic Injuries to the Teeth (3rd edn). Copenhagen: Munksgaard Publishers, 1993: pp. 151–177.
18. **Glendor U, Marcenes W, Andreasen JO**. Classification, epidemiology and etiology. In: Andreasen JO, Andreasen FM, Andersson L (eds), *Textbook and Color Atlas of Traumatic Injuries to the Teeth* (4th edn). Oxford: Blackwell, 2007. pp. 217–254.
19. IDCDA. *Application of the International Classification of Diseases to Dentistry and Stomatology IDCDA* (3rd edn). Geneva: WHO, 1995.

EXAMINATION AND DIAGNOSIS

20. **Andreasen FM, Andreasen JO, Tsukiboshi M**. Examination and diagnosis of dental injuries. In: Andreasen JO, Andreasen FM, Andersson L (eds), *Textbook and Color Atlas of Traumatic Injuries to the Teeth* (4th edn). Oxford: Blackwell, 2007. pp. 255–279.
21. **Andreasen FM, Andreasen JO**. Diagnosis of luxation injuries. The importance of standardized clinical, radiographic and photographic techniques in clinical investigations. *Endod Dent Traumatol* 1985;1:160–169.
22. **Bakland LK, Andreasen JO**. Examination of the dentally traumatized patient. *Calif Dent Ass J* 1996;24:35–44.
23. **Cohenca N, Simon JH, Roges R, Morag Y, Malfaz JM**. Clinical indications for digital imaging in dento-alveolar trauma. Part 1: traumatic injuries. *Dent Traumatol* 2007;23:95–104.

DIAGNOSIS OF PULPAL HEALING COMPLICATIONS

24. **Andreasen FM, Andreasen JO**. Luxation injuries of permanent teeth: general findings. In: Andreasen JO, Andreasen FM, Andersson L (eds), *Textbook and Color Atlas of Traumatic Injuries to the Teeth* (4th edn). Oxford: Blackwell, 2007. pp. 372–403.
25. **Andreasen FM, Yu Z, Thomsen ML, Andersen PK**. Occurrence of pulp canal obliteration after luxation injuries in the permanent dentition. *Endod Dent Traumatol* 1987;3:103–115.
26. **Robertson A, Andreasen FM, Bergenholtz G, Andreasen JO, Norén JG**. Incidence of pulp necrosis subsequent to pulp canal obliteration from trauma of permanent incisors. *J Endod* 1996;22:557–560.
27. **Andreasen FM**. Transient apical breakdown and its relation to color and sensibility changes after luxation injuries to teeth. *Endod Dent Traumatol* 1986;2:9–19.

DIAGNOSIS OF PERIODONTAL HEALING COMPLICATIONS

28. **Andreasen JO, Løvschall H**. Response of oral tissues to trauma. In: Andreasen JO, Andreasen FM, Andersson L (eds), *Textbook and Color Atlas of Traumatic Injuries to the Teeth* (4th edn). Oxford: Blackwell, 2007. pp. 62–113.
29. **Andreasen FM, Andreasen JO**. Root resorption following traumatic dental injuries. *Proc Finn Dent Soc* 1992;88:95–114.

30. **Andreasen FM, Andreasen JO**. Resorption and mineralization processes following root fracture of permanent incisors. *Endod Dent Traumatol* 1988;4:202–214.

TREATMENT PRIORITIES AFTER DENTAL TRAUMA

31. **Andreasen JO, Andreasen FM, Skeie A, Hjørting-Hansen E, Schwartz O**. Effect of treatment delay upon pulp and periodontal healing of traumatic dental injuries – a review article. *Dent Traumatol* 2002;18:116–128.

32. **Andreasen JO**. Fractures of the alveolar process of the jaw. A clinical and radiographic follow-up study. *Scand J Dent Res* 1970;78:263–272.

33. **Andreasen JO, Andreasen FM, Mèjare I, Cvek M**. Healing of 400 intra-alveolar root fractures. 2. Effect of treatment factors such as treatment delay, repositioning, splinting type period and antibiotics. *Dent Traumatol* 2004;20:203–211.

CROWN FRACTURE WITHOUT PULP EXPOSURE

34. **Andreasen FM, Andreasen JO**. Crown fractures. In: Andreasen JO, Andreasen FM, Andersson L (eds), *Textbook and Color Atlas of Traumatic Injuries to the Teeth* (4th edn). Oxford: Blackwell, 2007. pp. 280–305.

35. **Lauridsen EF, Hermann NV. Gerds TA, Ahrensburg SS, Andreasen JO**. Crown fractures, Part 1 – Healing complications of the pulp following crown fractures in the permanent incisors. *Dent Traumatol* 2011;27: in preparation.

36. **Lauridsen EF, Hermann NV, Gerds TA, Ahrensburg SS, Andreasen JO**. Crown fractures, Part 2 – Healing complications of the pulp in permanent incisors with crown fractures and concussion injury. *Dent Traumatol* 2011;27: in preparation.

37. **Lauridsen EF, Hermann NV. Gerds TA, Ahrensburg SS, Andreasen JO**. Crown fractures, Part 3 – Healing complications of the pulp in permanent incisors with crown fractures and subluxation injury. *Dent Traumatol* 2011;27: in preparation.

38. **Lauridsen EF, Hermann NV. Gerds TA, Ahrensburg SS, Andreasen JO**. Crown fractures, Part 4 – Healing complications of the pulp in permanent incisors following crown fractures with concurrent extrusion or lateral luxation injury. *Dent Traumatol* 2011;27: in preparation.

CROWN FRACTURE WITH PULP EXPOSURE

39. **Andreasen FM, Andreasen JO**. Crown fractures. In: Andreasen JO, Andreasen FM, Andersson L (eds), *Textbook and Color Atlas of Traumatic Injuries to the Teeth* (4th edn). Oxford: Blackwell, 2007. pp. 280–305.

40. **Lauridsen EF, Hermann NV. Gerds TA, Ahrensburg SS, Andreasen JO**. Crown fractures Part 1 – Healing complications of the pulp following crown fractures in the permanent incisors. *Dent Traumatol* 2011;27. In preparation.

41. **Lauridsen EF, Hermann NV. Gerds TA, Ahrensburg SS, Andreasen JO**. Crown fractures Part 2 – Healing complications of the pulp in permanent incisors with crown fractures and concussion injury. *Dent Traumatol* 2011;27: in preparation.

42. **Lauridsen EF, Hermann NV. Gerds TA, Ahrensburg SS, Andreasen JO**. Crown fractures Part 3 – Healing complications of the pulp in permanent incisors with crown fractures and subluxation injury. *Dent Traumatol* 2011;27: in preparation.

43. **Lauridsen EF, Hermann NV. Gerds TA, Ahrensburg SS, Andreasen JO**. Crown fractures Part 4 – Healing complications of the pulp in permanent incisors following crown fractures with concurrent extrusion or lateral luxation injury. *Dent Traumatol* 2011;27: in preparation.

44. **Ravn JJ**. Follow-up study of permanent incisors with complicated crown fractures after acute trauma. *Scand J Dent Res* 1982;90:363–372.

45. **Cvek M**. A clinical report on partial pulpotomy and capping with calcium hydroxide in permanent incisors with complicated crown fracture. *J Endod* 1978;4:232–237.

46. **Fuks AB, Bielak S, Chosak A**. Clinical and radiographic assessment of direct pulp capping and pulpotomy in young permanent teeth. *Pediatr Dent* 1982;4:240–244.

47. **Cvek M**. Partial pulpotomy in crown-fractures incisors – results 3 to 15 years after treatment. *Acta Stomatologica Croatica* 1993;27:167–173.

48. **Cvek M**. Endodontic management and the use of calcium hydroxide in traumatized permanent teeth. In: Andreasen JO, Andreasen FM, Andersson L (eds), *Textbook and Color Atlas of Traumatic Injuries to the Teeth* (4th edn). Oxford: Blackwell, 2007. pp. 598–658.

CROWN-ROOT FRACTURE

49. **Andreasen JO, Andreasen FM**. Crown-root fractures. In: Andreasen JO, Andrasen FM, Andersson L (eds), *Textbook and Color Atlas of Traumatic Injuries to the Teeth* (4th edn). Oxford: Blackwell, 2007. pp. 314–366.

50. **Flores MT, Andersson L, Andreasen JO, Bakland LK, Malmgren B, Barnett F, Bourguignon C, DiAngelis A, Hicks L, Sigurdsson A, Trope M, Tsukiboshi M, von Arx T**. Guidelines for the management of traumatic dental injuries. I. Fractures and luxations of permanent teeth. *Dent Traumatol* 2007;23:66–71.

51. **Bessermann M, Andreasen JO, Ahrensburg SS, Selmer U**. Long term prognosis of anterior crown-root fractured teeth treated by orthodontic and/or surgical exposure of the fracture site. *Dent Traumatol* 2010;26: in preparation.

52. **Kahnberg K-E**. Surgical extrusion of root fractured teeth – a follow-up study of two surgical methods. *Endod Dent Traumatol* 1988;45–89.

53. **Kahnberg K-E, Warfvinge J, Birgersson B**. Intraalveolar transplantation (I). The use of autologous bone transplants in the periapical region. *Int J Oral Surg* 1982;11:372–379.

54. **Kahnberg K-E**. Intraalveolar transplantation of teeth with crown-root fractures. *J Oral Surg* 1985;43:38–42.

55. **Warfvinge J, Kahnberg K-E**. Intraalveolar transplantation of teeth. IV. Endodontic considerations. *Swed Dent J* 1989;13:229–233.

56. **Tegsjö U, Valerius-Olsson H, Olgart K**. Intra-alveolar transplantation of teeth with cervical root fractures. *Swed Dent J* 1978;2:73–82.

57. **Caliska MK, Türrün M, Gomel M**. Surgical extrusion of crown-root-fractured teeth: a clinical review. *Int Endod J* 1999;32:146–151.

ROOT FRACTURE

58. **Andreasen FM, Andreasen JO, Cvek M**. Root fractures. In: Andreasen JO, Andreasen FM, Andersson L (eds), *Textbook and Color Atlas of Traumatic Injuries to the Teeth* (4th edn). Oxford: Blackwell, 2007. pp. 337–371.

59. **Andreasen JO, Andreasen FM, Mejàre I, Cvek M**. Healing of 400 intra-alveolar root fractures. 1. Effect of pre-injury and injury factors such as sex, age, stage of root development, fracture type, location of fracture and severity of disclocation. *Dent Traumatol* 2004;20:192–202.

60. **Andreasen JO, Andreasen FM, Mèjare I, Cvek M**. Healing of 400 intra-alveolar root fractures. 2. Effect of treatment factors such as treatment delay, repositioning, splinting type period and antibiotics. *Dent Traumatol* 2004;20:203–211.

61. **Flores MT, Andersson L, Andreasen JO, Bakland LK, Malmgren B, Barnett F, Bourguignon C, DiAngelis A, Hicks L, Sigurdsson A, Trope M, Tsukiboshi M, von Arx T**. Guidelines for the management of traumatic dental injuries. I. Fractures and luxations of permanent teeth. *Dent Traumatol* 2007;23:66–71.

62. **Cvek M, Mejàre I, Andreasen JO**. Healing and prognosis of teeth with intraalveolar fractures involving the cervical part of the root. *Dent Traumatol* 2002;18:57–65.

63. **Andreasen JO, Hjørting-Hansen E**. Intraalveolar root fractures: radiographic and histologic study of 50 cases. *J Oral Surg* 1967; 25:414–426.

64. **Cvek M**. Treament of non-vital permanent incisors with calcium hydroxide. IV. Periodontal healing and closure of the root canal in the coronal fragment of teeth with intra-alveolar fracture and vital apical fragment. *Odont Rev* 1974;25:239–245.

65. **Cvek M, Mèjare I, Andreasen JO**. Conservative endodontic treatment of teeth fractured in the middle or apical part of the root. *Dent Traumatol* 2004;20:261–269.

66. **Andreasen FM, Andreasen JO, Bayer T**. Prognosis of root fractured permanent incisors – prediction of healing modalities. *Endod Dent Traumatol* 1989;5:11–22.

67. **Andreasen FM, Andreasen JO**. Resorption and mineralization processes following root fracture of permanent incisors. *Endod Dent Traumatol* 1988;4:202–214.

68. **Cvek M, Tsilingaridis G, Andreasen JO**. Survival of 534 incisors after intra-alveolar root fracture in patients aged 7–17 years. *Dent Traumatol* 2008;24:379–387.

ALVEOLAR PROCESS FRACTURE

69. **Andreasen JO**. Injuries to the supporting bone. In: Andreasen JO, Andreasen FM, Andersson L (eds), *Textbook and Color Atlas of Traumatic Injuries to the Teeth* (4th edn). Oxford: Blackwell, 2007. pp. 489–515.

70. **Andreasen JO, Ahrensburg SS, Hillerup S, Kofod T, Schwartz O**. Alveolar fractures in the permanent dentition. Part 1. Epidemiology, etiology and pathogenesis. An analysis of 340 cases involving 800 teeth. *Dent Traumatol* 2011;27: in preparation.

71. **Andreasen JO, Ahrensburg SS, Hillerup S, Kofod T, Schwartz O**. Alveolar fractures in the permanent dentition. Part 2. A clinical prospective study of 83 cases involving 197 teeth. Effect of preinjury and injury factors upon healing complications. *Dent Traumatol* 2011;27: in preparation.

72. **Andreasen JO, Ahrensburg SS, Hillerup S, Kofod T, Schwartz O**. Alveolar fractures in the permanent dentition. Part 3. A clinical prospective study of 83 cases involving 197 teeth. Effect of treatment factors upon healing complications. *Dent Traumatol* 2011;27: in preparation.

73. **Flores MT, Andersson L, Andreasen JO, Bakland LK, Malmgren B, Barnett F, Bourguignon C, DiAngelis A, Hicks L, Sigurdsson A, Trope M, Tsukiboshi M, von Arx T**. Guidelines for the management of traumatic dental injuries. I. Fractures and luxations of permanent teeth. *Dent Traumatol* 2007;23:66–71.

CONCUSSION

74. **Andreasen FM, Andreasen JO**. Concussion and subluxation. In: Andreasen JO, Andreasen FM, Andersson L (eds), *Textbook and Color Atlas of Traumatic Injuries to the Teeth* (4th edn). Oxford: Blackwell, 2007. pp. 404–410.

75. **Flores MT, Andersson L, Andreasen JO, Bakland LK, Malmgren B, Barnett F, Bourguignon C, DiAngelis A, Hicks L, Sigurdsson A, Trope M, Tsukiboshi M, von Arx T**. Guidelines for the management of traumatic dental injuries. I. Fractures and luxations of permanent teeth. *Dent Traumatol* 2007;23:66–71.

76. **Andreasen FM, Vestergaard Pedersen B**. Prognosis of luxated permanent teeth – the development of pulp necrosis. *Endod Dent Traumatol* 1985;1:207–220.

77. **Herman NV, Andreasen JO, Andreasen FM, Ahrensburg SS**. Healing complications following concussion injury in the permanent dentition. *Dent Traumatol* 2011;27: in preparation.

SUBLUXATION

78. **Andreasen FM, Andreasen JO**. Concussion and subluxation. In: Andreasen JO, Andreasen FM, Andersson L (eds), *Textbook and Color Atlas of Traumatic Injuries to the Teeth* (4th edn). Oxford: Blackwell, 2007. pp. 404–410.

79. **Flores MT, Andersson L, Andreasen JO, Bakland LK, Malmgren B, Barnett F, Bourguignon C, DiAngelis A, Hicks L, Sigurdsson A, Trope M, Tsukiboshi M, von Arx T**. Guidelines for the management of traumatic dental injuries. I. Fractures and luxations of permanent teeth. *Dent Traumatol* 2007;23:66–71.

80 **Andreasen FM, Vestergaard Pedersen B**. Prognosis of luxated permanent teeth – the development of pulp necrosis. *Endod Dent Traumatol* 1985;1:207–220.

81. **Lauridsen EF, Hermann NV, Gerds TA, Ahrensburg SS, Andreasen JO**. Crown fractures Part 3 – Healing complications of the pulp in permanent incisors with crown fractures and subluxation injury. *Dent Traumatol* 2011;27: in preparation.

82. **Herman NV, Andreasen JO, Andreasen F, Ahrensburg SS**. Healing complications following subluxation injury in the permanent dentition. *Dent Traumatol* 2011;27; in preparation.

EXTRUSIVE LUXATION

83. **Andreasen FM, Andreasen JO**. Extrusive luxation and lateral luxation. In: Andreasen JO, Andreasen FM, Andersson L (eds), *Textbook and Color Atlas of Traumatic Injuries to the Teeth* (4th edn). Oxford: Blackwell, 2007. pp. 411–427.

84. **Flores MT, Andersson L, Andreasen JO, Bakland LK, Malmgren B, Barnett F, Bourguignon C, DiAngelis A, Hicks L, Sigurdsson A, Trope M, Tsukiboshi M, von Arx T**. Guidelines for the management of traumatic dental injuries. I. Fractures and luxations of permanent teeth. *Dent Traumatol* 2007;23:66–71.

85. **Andreasen FM, Vestergaard Pedersen B**. Prognosis of luxated permanent teeth – the development of pulp necrosis. *Endod Dent Traumatol* 1985;1:207–220.

86. **Andreasen FM, Yu Z, Thomsen BL**. The relationship between pulpal dimensions and the development of pulp necrosis after luxation injuries in the permanent dentition. *Endod Dent Traumatol* 1986;2:90–98.

87. **Andreasen FM, Yu Z, Thomsen BL, Anderson PK**. Occurrence of pulp canal obliteration after luxation in the permanent dentition. *Endod Dent Traumatol* 1987;23:103–115.

88. **Lauridsen EF, Hermann NV, Gerds TA, Ahrensburg SS, Andreasen JO**. Crown fractures Part 4 – healing complications of the pulp in permanent incisors following crown fractures with concurrent extrusion or lateral luxation injury. *Dent Traumatol* 2011;27: in preparation.

89. **Herman NV, Andreasen JO, Andreasen F, Ahrensburg SS**. Healing complications following extrusive luxation injury in the permanent dentition. *Dent Traumatol* 2011;27: in preparation.

90. **Lee R, Barrett, EJ, Kenny DJ**. Clinical outcomes for permanent incisor luxations in a pediatric population. II. Extrusions. *Dent Traumatol* 2003;19:274–279.

LATERAL LUXATION

91. **Andreasen FM, Andreasen JO**. Extrusive luxation and lateral luxation. In: Andreasen JO, Andreasen FM, Andersson L (eds), *Textbook and Color Atlas of Traumatic Injuries to the Teeth* (4th edn). Oxford: Blackwell, 2007. pp. 411–427.

92. **Flores MT, Andersson L, Andreasen JO, Bakland LK, Malmgren B, Barnett F, Bourguignon C, DiAngelis A, Hicks L, Sigurdsson A, Trope M, Tsukiboshi M, von Arx T**. Guidelines for the management of traumatic dental

injuries. I. Fractures and luxations of permanent teeth. *Dent Traumatol* 2007;23:66–71.

93. **Andreasen FM, Vestergaard Pedersen B**. Prognosis of luxated permanent teeth – the development of pulp necrosis. *Endod Dent Traumatol* 1985;1:207–220.

94. **Andreasen FM, Yu Z, Thomsen BL**. The relationship between pulpal dimensions and the development of pulp necrosis after luxation injuries in the permanent dentition. *Endod Dent Traumatol* 1986;2:90–98.

95. **Andreasen FM, Yu Z, Thomsen BL, Anderson PK**. Occurrence of pulp canal obliteration after luxation in the permanent dentition. *Endod Dent Traumatol* 1987;23:103–115.

96. **Lauridsen EF, Hermann NV, Gerds TA, Ahrensburg SS, Andreasen JO**. Crown fractures Part 4 – healing complications of the pulp in permanent incisors following crown fractures with concurrent extrusion or lateral luxation injury. *Dent Traumatol* 2011;27: in preparation

97. **Elena C, Ferrazzini P, von Arx T**. Pulp and periodontal healing of laterally luxated permanent teeth: results after 4 years. *Dent Traumatol* 2008;24:658–662.

98. **Nikoui M, Kenny DJ, Barrett EJ**. Clinical outcomes for permanent incisor luxations in a pediatric population.III. Lateral luxation. *Dent Traumatol* 2003;19:280–285.

99. **Herman NV, Andreasen JO, Andreasen F, Ahrensburg SS**. Healing complications following lateral luxation injury in the permanent dentition. *Dent Traumatol* 2011;27: in preparation.

INTRUSIVE LUXATION

100. **Andreasen FM, Andreasen JO**. Intrusive luxation and lateral luxation. In: Andreasen JO, Andreasen FM, Andersson L (eds), *Textbook and Color Atlas of Traumatic Injuries to the Teeth* (4th edn). Oxford: Blackwell, 2007. pp. 428–443.

101. **Flores MT, Andersson L, Andreasen JO, Bakland LK, Malmgren B, Barnett F, Bourguignon C, DiAngelis A, Hicks L, Sigurdsson A, Trope M, Tsukiboshi M, von Arx T**. Guidelines for the management of traumatic dental injuries. I. Fractures and luxations of permanent teeth. *Dent Traumatol* 2007;23:66–71.

102. **Andreasen JO, Bakland LK, Matras R, Andreasen FM**. Traumatic intrusion of permanent teeth. Part 1. An epidemiological study of 216 intruded permanent teeth. *Dent Traumatol* 2006;22:83–89.

103. **Andreasen JO, Bakland LK, Matras R, Andreasen FM**. Traumatic intrusion of permanent teeth. Part 2. A clinical

study of the effect of preinjury and injury factors (such as sex, age, stage of root development, tooth location, and extent of injury including number of intruded teeth) on 140 intruded permanent teeth. *Dent Traumatol* 2006;22:90–98.

104. **Andreasen JO, Bakland LK, Matras R, Andreasen FM**. Traumatic intrusion of permanent teeth. Part 3. A clinical study of the effect of treatment variables such as treatment delay, method of repositioning, type of splint, length of splinting and antibiotics on 140 teeth. *Dent Traumatol* 2006;22:99–111.

105. **Ebeleseder KA, Santler G, Glockner K, Hulla H, Pertl C, Quenhenberger F**. An analysis of 58 traumatically intruded and surgically extruded permanent teeth. *Endod Dent Traumatol* 2000;16:34–39.

106. **Kinirons MJ, Sutcliffe J**. Traumatically intruded permanent incisors: a study of treatment and outcome. *Br Dent J* 1991;170:144–146.

107. **Al-Badri S, Kinirons M, Cole BOI, Welbury RR**. Factors afflicting resorption in traumatically intruded permanent incisors in children. *Dent Traumatol* 2002;18:73–76.

108. **Humphrey JM, Kenny DJ, Barrett EJ**. Clinical outcomes for permanent incisor luxations in a pediatric population. I. Intrusions. *Dent Traumatol* 2003;19:266–273.

109. **Chaushu S, Shapiro J, Heling J, Becker A**. Emergency orthodontic treatment after the traumatic intrusive luxation of maxillary incisors. *Am J Orthod Dentofacial Orthop* 2004;126:162–172.

110. **Wigen TI, Agnalt R, Jacobsen I**. Intrusive luxation of permanent incisors in Norwegians aged 6–17 years: a retrospective study of treatment and outcome. *Dent Traumatol* 2008;24:612–618.

AVULSION

111. **Andreasen FM, Andreasen JO**. Avulsions. In: Andreasen JO, Andreasen FM, Andersson L (eds), *Textbook and Color Atlas of Traumatic Injuries to the Teeth* (4th edn). Oxford: Blackwell, 2007. pp. 444–488.

112. **Flores MT, Andersson L, Andreasen JO, Bakland LK, Malmgren B, Barnett F, Bourguignon C, DiAngelis A, Hicks L, Sigurdsson A, Trope M, Tsukiboshi M, von Arx T**. Guidelines for the management of traumatic dental injuries. II. Avulsion of permanent teeth. *Dent Traumatol* 2007; 23: 130–136.

113. **Coccia CT**. A clinical investigation of root resorption rates in reimplanted young permanent incisors: a five-year study. *J Endod* 1980;6:413–420.

114. **Andreasen JO, Jensen SS, Sae-Lim V**. The role of antibiotics in preventing healing complications after traumatic dental injuries: a literature review. *Endod Topics* 2006;14:80–92.

115. **Hammarström L, Blomlöf L, Feiglin B, Andersson L, Lindskog S**. Replantation of teeth and antibiotic treatment. *Endod Dent Traumatol* 1986;2:51–57.

116. **Cvek M, Cleaton-Jones P, Austin J, Lownie J, Kling M, Fatti P**. Effect of topical application of doxycycline on pulp revascularization and periodontal healing in reimplanted monkey incisors. *Endod Dent Traumatol* 1990;6:170–176.

117. **Cvek M, Cleaton-Jones P, Austin J, King M, Lownie J, Fatti P**. Pulp revascularization in reimplanted immature monkey incisors – predictability and the effect of antibiotic systemic prophylaxis. *Endod Dent Traumatol* 1990;6:157–169.

118. **Ritter AL, Ritter AV, Murrah V, Sigurdsson A, Trope M**. Pulp revascularization of replanted immature dog teeth after treatment with minocycline and doxycycline assessed by laser Doppler flowmetry, radiography, and histology. *Dent Traumatol* 2004;20:75–84.

119. **Sae-Lim V, Wang CY, Trope M**. Effect of systemic tetracycline and amoxicillin on inflammatory root resorption of replanted dogs' teeth. *Endod Dent Traumatol* 1998:14:216–220.

120. **Yanpiset K, Trope M**. Pulp revascularization of replanted immature dog teeth after different treatment methods. *Endod Dent Traumatol* 2000;16:211–217.

121. **Cvek M, Granath LE, Hollender L**. Treatment of non-vital permanent incisors with calcium hydroxide. III. Variation of occurrence of ankylosis of reimplanted teeth with duration of extra-alveolar period and storage enviroment. *Odont Rev* 1974;25: 43–56.

122. **Andreasen JO, Borum MK, Ahrensburg SS, Andreasen FM**. Replantation of 400 traumatically avulsed permanent incisors VI – endodontic procedures related to periodontal healing or progression of root resorption. *Dent Traumatol* 2010;26: in preparation.

123. **Andreasen JO, Borum M, Jacobsen HL, Andreasen FM**. Replantation of 400 traumatically avulsed permanent incisors. I. Diagnosis of healing complications. *Endod Dent Traumatol* 1995;11:51–58.

124. **Andreasen JO, Borum M, Jacobsen HL, Andreasen FM**. Replantation of 400 avulsed permanent incisors. II. Factors related to pulp healing. *Endod Dent Traumatol* 1995;11:59–68.

125. **Andreasen JO, Borum M, Jacobsen HL, Andreasen FM**. Replantation of 400 avulsed permanent incisors. III. Factors related to root growth after replantation. *Endod Dent Traumatol* 1995;11:69–75.

126. **Andreasen JO, Borum M, Jacobsen HL, Andreasen FM**. Replantation of 400 avulsed permanent incisors. IV. Factors related to periodontal ligament healing. *Endod Dent Traumatol* 1995;11:76–89.

127. **Andreasen JO, Borum MK, Loft Jacobsen H, Ahrensburg SS, Andreasen FM**. Replantation of 400 traumatically avulsed permanent incisors V – preinjury and injury factors related to progression of root resorption. *Dent Traumatol* 2010;26: in preparation.

128. **Andreasen JO**. Periodontal healing after replantation of traumatically avulsed human teeth. Assessment by mobility testing and radiography. *Acta Odontol Scand* 1975;33:325–335.

129. **Andreasen JO, Jensen L, Ahrensburg SS**. Relationship between calcium hydroxide pH levels in the root canals and periodontal healing after replantation of avulsed teeth. *Endod Topics* 2006;14:93–101.

130. **Kling M, Cvek M, Mejare I**. Rate and predictability of pulp revascularization in therapeutically reimplanted permanent incisors. *Endod Dent Traumatol* 1986;2:83–89.

131. **Mackie IC, Worthington HV**. An investigation of replantation of traumatically avulsed permanent incisor teeth. *Br Dent J* 1992;172:17–20.

132. **Schatz JP, Hausherr C, Joho JP**. A retrospective clinical and radiologic study of teeth re-implanted following traumatic avulsion. *Endod Dent Traumatol* 1995;11:235–239.

133. **Barrett EJ, Kenny DJ**. Survival of avulsed permanent maxillary incisors in children following delayed replantation. *Endod Dent Traumatol* 1997;13:269–275.

134. **Sae-Lim V, Yuen KW**. An evaluation of after-office-hour dental trauma in Singapore. *Endod Dent Traumatol* 1997;13:164–170.

135. **Ebeseleder KA, Friehs S, Ruda C, Pertl C, Glockner K, Hulla H**. A study of replanted permanent teeth in different age groups. *Endod Dent Traumatol* 1998;14:274–278.

136. **Kinirons MJ, Boyd DH, Gregg TA**. Inflammatory and replacement resorption in reimplanted permanent incisors teeth: a study of the characteristics of 84 teeth. *Endod Dent Traumatol* 1999;15:269–272.

137. **Boyd DH, Kinirons MJ, Gregg TA**. A prospective study of factors affecting survival of replanted permanent incisors in children. *Int J Paediatric Dent* 2000;10:200–205.

138. **Kinirons MJ, Gregg TA, Welbury RR, Cole BO**. Variations in the presenting and treatment features in reimplantated permanent incisors in children and their effect on the prevalence of root resorption. *Br Dent J* 2000;189:263–266.

139. **Donaldson M, Kinirons MJ**. Factors affecting the onset of resorption in avulsed and replanted incisors teeth in children. *Dent Traumatol* 2001;17:205–209.

140. **Chappuis V, von Arx T**. Replantation of 45 avulsed permanent teeth: a 1 year follow-up study. *Dent Traumatol* 2005;21:289–296.

141. **Pohl Y, Filippi A, Kirschner H**. Results after replantation of avulsed permanent teeth. I. Endodontic considerations. *Dent Traumatol* 2005;21:80–92.

142. **Pohl Y, Filippi A, Kirschner H**. Results after replantation of avulsed permanent teeth. II. Periodontal healing and the role of physiologic storage and antiresorptive-regenerative therapy. *Dent Traumatol* 2005;21:93–101.

143. **Pohl Y, Filippi A, Kirschner H**. Results after replantation of avulsed permanent teeth. III. Tooth loss and survival analysis. *Dent Traumatol* 2005;21:102–110.

144. **Stewart CJ, Elledge RO, Kinirons MJ, Welbury RR**. Factors affecting the timing of pulp extirpation in a sample of 66 replanted avulsed teeth in children and adolescents. *Dent Traumatol* 2008;24:625–627.

145. **Soares AJ, Gomes BPFA, Zaia AA, Ferraz CCR, Souza-Filho FJ**. Relationship between clinical-radiographic evaluation and outcome of teeth replantation. *Dent Traumatol* 2008;24:183–188.

INJURIES TO THE PRIMARY DENTITION

146. **Flores MT, Holan G, Borum M, Andreasen JO**. Injuries to the Primary Dentition. In: Andreasen JO, Andreasen FM, Andersson L (eds), *Textbook and Color Atlas of Traumatic Injuries to the Teeth* (4th edn). Oxford: Blackwell, 2007. pp. 516–541.

147. **Andreasen JO, Flores MT**. Injuries to developing teeth. In: Andreasen JO, Andreasen FM, Andersson L (eds), *Textbook and Color Atlas of Traumatic Injuries to the Teeth* (4th edn). Oxford: Blackwell, 2007. pp. 542–576.

148. **Flores MT, Malmgren B, Andersson L, Andreasen JO, Bakland A, Trope M, Tsukiboshi M, von Arx T**. Guidelines for the management of traumatic dental injuries. III Primary teeth. *Dent Traumatol* 2007;23:196–202.

149. **Borum MK, Andreasen JO**. Sequelae of trauma to primary maxillary incisors. I. Complications in the primary dentition. *Endod Dent Traumatol* 1998;14:31–44.

150. **Andreasen JO, Sundström B, Ravn JJ**. The effect of traumatic injuries to primary teeth on their permanent successors. I. A clinical and histologic study of 117 injured permanent teeth. *Scand J Dent Res* 1971;79:219–283.

151. **Andreasen JO, Ravn JJ**. The effect of traumatic injuries to primary teeth on their permanent successors. II. A clinical and radiographic follow-up study of 213 injured teeth. *Scand J Dent Res* 1971;79:284–294.

152. **Andreasen JO, Ravn JJ**. Enamel changes in permanent teeth after trauma of their primary predecessors. *Scand J Dent Res* 1973;81:203–209.

153. **Selliseth N-E**. The significance of traumatised primary incisors on the development and eruption of permanent teeth. *Eur Orthodont Dent Soc* 1970;46:443–459.

154. **Ben Bassat Y, Brin I, Fuks A, Zilberman Y**. Effect of trauma to the primary incisors on permanent successors in different developmental stages. *Pediatr Dent* 1985;7:37–40.

155. **Zilberman Y, Ben Bassat Y, Lustmann J**. Effect of trauma to primary incisors on root development to their permanent successors. *Pediatr Dent* 1986;8:289–293.

156. **von Arx T**. Traumatologie im Milchgebiss (I). Klinische und therapeutische Aspekte. *Schweiz Monatsschr Zahnmed* 1990;100: 1195–1204.

157. **von Arx T**. Traumatologie im Milchgebiss (II). Langzeitergebnisse sowie Auswirkungen auf das Milchgebiss und die bleibende Dentition. *Schweiz Monatsschr Zahnmed* 1991;101:57–68.

158. **Colak I, Markovic D, Petrovic B, Peric T, Milenkovic A**. A retrospective study of intrusive injuries in primary dentition. *Dent Traumatol* 2009;25:605–610.

SOFT TISSUE INJURIES

159. **Andersson L, Andreasen JO**. Soft tissue injuries. In: Andreasen JO, Andreasen FM, Andersson L (eds), *Textbook and Color Atlas of Traumatic injuries to the Teeth* (4th edn). Oxford: Blackwell, Munksgaard, 2007. pp. 577–597.

160. **Lindfors J**. A comparison of an antimicrobial wound cleanser to normal saline in reduction of bioburden and its effect on wound healing. *Ostomy Wound Manag* 2004;50:28–41.

161. **Peterson JA, Cardo VA, Stratigos GT**. An examination of antibiotic prophylaxis in oral and maxillofacial surgery. *J Oral Surg* 1970;28:753–759.

162. **Valente JH, Forti RJ, Freundlich LF, Zandieh SO,Crain EF**. Wound irrigation in children: saline solution or tap water? *Ann Emerg Med* 2003;41:609–616.

163. **Herford AS**. Early repair of avulsive facial wounds secondary to trauma using interpolation flaps. *J Oral Maxillofac Surg* 2004;62: 959–965.

164. **Rhee ST, Colville C, Buchman SR**. Conservative management of large avulsion of the lip and local landmarks. *Pediatr Emerg Care* 2004;20:40–42.

165. **Schockledge RR, Mackie IC**. Oral soft tissue trauma: gingival degloving. *Endod Dent Traumatol* 1996;11:109–111.

166. **Al Melh M, Andersson L, Behbehani E**. Reduction of pain from needlestick in the oral mucosa by topical anesthetics: a comparative study between lidocaine/prilocaine and benzocaine. *J Clin Dent* 2006; 16:53–56.

167. **Al Melh MA, Andersson L**. Comparison of topical anesthetics (EMLA/Oraqix vs Benzocaine) on pain experienced during palatal needle injection. *Oral Surg Oral Med Oral Pathol Oral Radiol Endod* 2007;103:e16–20. Epub 2007, Feb 27.

168. **Al Asfour A, Al Melh M, Andersson L, Joseph B**. Healing pattern of experimental soft tissue laceration after application of novel topical anesthetic agents – an experimental study in rabbits. *Dent Traumatol* 2008;24:27–31.

169. **Mark DG, Granquist EJ**. Are prophylactic oral antibiotics indicated for the treatment of intraoral wounds? *Ann Emerg Med* 2008;52:368–372.

170. **Cummings P, Del Beccaro MA**. Antibiotics to prevent infection of simple wounds: a meta-analysis of randomized studies. *Am J Emerg Med* 1995;13:396–400.

171. **Holger JS, Wandersee SE, Hale DB**. Cosmetic outcome of facial lacerations repaired with tissue adhesive, absorbable and non-absorbable sutures. *Am J Emerg Med* 2004;22:254–257.

172. **Farion K, Osmond MH, Hartling L**. Tissue adhesives for traumatic lacerations in children and adults. *Cochrane Database of Systematic Reviews* 2002(3).

173. **Medeiros I, Saconato H**. Antibiotic prophylaxis for mammalian bites. *Cochrane Database of Systematic Reviews* 2001(2).

SPLINTING

174. **Oikarinen KS**. Splinting of traumatized teeth. In: Andreasen JO, Andreasen FM, Andersson (eds), *Textbook and Color Atlas of Traumatic Injuries to the Teeth* (4th edn). Oxford: Blackwell, Munksgaard, 2007. pp. 842–851.

175. **Mandel U, Viidik A**. Effect of splinting on the mechanical and histological properties of the healing periodontal ligament in the vervet monkey (*Cercopithecus aethiops*). *Arch Oral Biol* 1989;34:209–217.

176. **Andreasen JO**. The effect of splinting upon periodontal and pulpal healing after replantation of permanent incisors in monkeys. *Acta Odontal Scand* 1975;33:313–323.

177. **Kristerson L, Andreasen JO**. The effect of splinting upon periodontal and pulpal healing after autotransplantation of mature and immature permanent incisors in monkeys. *Int J Oral Surg* 1983;12: 239–249.

178. **Oikarinen K**. Functional fixation for traumatically luxated teeth. *Endod Dent Traumatol* 1987;3:224–228.

179. **Oikarinen K**. Comparison of the flexibility of various splinting methods for tooth fixation. *J Oral Maxillofac Surg* 1988;17:225–227.

180. **Oikarinen K**. Tooth splinting: a review of the literature and consideration of the versality of a wire-composite splint. *Endod Dent Traumatol* 1990;6:237–250.

181. **Oikarinen K, Andreasen JO, Andreasen FM**. Rigidity of various fixation methods used as dental splints. *Endod Dent Traumatol* 1992;8:113–119.

182. **Berthold C, Thaler A, Petschelt A**. Rigidity of commonly used dental trauma splints. *Dent Traumatol* 2009;25:248–255.

183. **Andersson L, Lindskog S, Blomlof L, Hedstrom KG, Hammarstrom L**. Effect of masticatory stimulation on dentoalveolar ankylosis after experimental tooth replantation. *Endod Dent Traumatol* 1985;1:13–16.

184. **von Arx T, Filippi A, Buser D**. Splinting of traumatized teeth with a new device: TTS (Titanium Trauma Splint). *Dent Traumatol* 2001;17:180–184.

185. **von Arx T, Filippi A, Lussi A**. Comparison of a new dental trauma splint device (TTS) with three commonly used splinting techniques. *Dent Traumatol* 2001;17: 266–274.

186. **Stellini E, Avesani S, Mazzoleni S, Favero L**. Laboratory comparison of a titanium trauma splint with three conventional ones for the treatment of dental trauma. *Eur J Paediatr Dent* 2005;6:191–196.

187. **Kahler B, Heithersay GS**. An evidence-based appraisal of splinting luxated, avulsed and root-fractured teeth. *Dent Traumatol* 2008;24:2–10.

ENDODONTIC CONSIDERATIONS IN DENTAL TRAUMA

188. **Bakland LK**. New endodontic procedures using mineral trioxide aggregate (MTA) for teeth with traumatic Injuries. In: Andreasen JO, Andreasen FM, Andersson L. *Textbook and Color Atlas of Traumatic Injuries to the Teeth*, (4th edn). Copenhagen: Munksgaard, 1993. pp. 658–668.

189. **Cvek M.** Endodontic management and the use of calcium hydroxide in traumatized permanent teeth. In: Andreasen JO, Andreasen FM, Andersson L. *Textbook and Color Atlas of Traumatic Injuries to the Teeth* (4th edn). Copenhagen: Munksgaard, 2007. pp. 598–668.

190. **Andersen M, Lund A, Andreasen JO, Andreasen FM**. In vitro solidity of human pulp tissue in calcium hydroxite and sodium hypochlorite. *Endod Dent Traumatol* 1992;8:104–108.

191. **Andreasen JO, Farik B, Munksgaard EC**. Long-term calcium hydroxide as a root canal dressing may increase risk of root fracture. *Dent Traumatol* 2002;18:134–137.

192. **Cvek M**. Prognosis of luxated non-vital maxillary incisors treated with calcium hydroxite and filled with gutta-percha. *Endod Dent Traumatol* 1992;8:45–55.

193. **Torabinejad M, Watson TF, Pitt Ford TR**. The sealing ability of a mineral trioxide aggregate as a retrograde root filling material. *J Endod* 1993;19:591–595.

194. **Torabinejad M, Hong CU, Pitt Ford TR**. Physical and chemical properties of a new root end filling material. *J Endod* 1995;21:349–353.

195. **Pitt Ford TR, Torabinejad M, Abedi HR, Bakland LK, Kariyawasam SP**. Mineral trioxide aggregate as a pulp capping material. *J Am Dent Ass* 1996;127:1491–1494.

196. **Torabinejad M, Chivian N**. Clinical applications of mineral trioxide aggregate. *J Endod* 1999;25:197–205.

197. **Faraco IM Jr, Holland R**. Response of the pulp of dogs to capping with mineral trioxide aggregate or a calcium hydroxide cement. *Dent Traumatol* 2001;17:163–166.

198. **Tziafas D, Pantelidou O, Alvanou A, Belibasakis G, Papadimitriou S**. The dentinogenic effect of mineral trioxide aggregate (MTA) in short-term capping experiments. *Int Endod J* 2002;35:245–254.

199. **Nair PN, Duncan HF, Pitt Ford TR, Luder HU**. Histological, ultrastructural and quantitative investigations on the response of healthy human pulps to experimental capping with Mineral Trioxide Aggregate: a randomized controlled trial. *Int Endod J* 2009;42:422–444.

200. **Olsson H, Petersson K, Rohlin M**. Formation of a hard tissue barrier after pulp cappings in humans. A systematic review. *Int Endod J* 2006;39:429–442.

201. **Shabahang S, Torabinejad M**. Treatment of teeth with open apices using mineral trioxide aggregate.

Pract Periodont Aesthet Dent 2000;12:315–320.

202. **Giuliani V, Baccetti T, Pace R, Pagavino G**. The use of MTA in teeth with necrotic pulps and open apices. *Dent Traumatol* 2002;18:217–221.

203. **Menezes R, Bramante CM, Letra A, Carvalho VG, Garcia RB**. Histologic evaluation of pulpotomies in dog using two types of mineral trioxide aggregate and regular and white Portland cements as wound dressings. *Oral Surg Oral Med Oral Pathol Oral Radiol Endod* 2004;98:276–279.

204. **Torabinejad M, Pitt Ford TR, McKendry DJ, Abedi HR, Miller DA, Kariywasam SP**. Histologic assessment of mineral trioxide aggregate as a root-end filling material in monkeys. *J Endod* 1997;23: 225–228.

205. **Faraco IM Jr, Holland R**. Response of the pulp dogs to capping with Mineral Trioxide Aggregate or a calcium hydroxide cement. *Dent Traumatol* 2001;17:163–166.

206. **Shabahang S, Torabinejad M, Boyne PP, Abedi H, McMillan P**. A comparative study of root-end induction using osteogenic protein-1, calcium hydroxide, and mineral trioxide aggregate in dogs. *J Endod* 1999;25:1–5.

DECORONATION OF ANKYLOSED TEETH IN ADOLESCENTS

207. **Malmgren B, Malmgren O, Andreasen JO**. Alveolar bone development after decoronation of ankylosed teeth. *Endod Topics* 2006;14:35–40.

208. **Malmgren B, Cvek M, Lundberg M, Frykholm A**. Surgical treatment of ankylosed and infrapositioned reimplanted incisors in adolescents. *Scand J Dent Res* 1984;92:391–399.

209. **Malmgren B, Malmgren O**. Rate of infraposition of reimplanted ankylosed incisors related to age and growth in children and adolescents. *Dent Traumatol* 2002:18:28–36.

210. **Malmgren B**. Decoronation: how, why and when? *J Cal Dent Assoc* 2000:28:846–854.

PREDICTORS FOR HEALING COMPLICATIONS

211. **Andreasen JO, Vinding TR, SS Ahrensburg**. Predictors for healing complications in the permanent dentition after dental trauma. *Endod Topics* 2006;14:20–27.

212. The Dental Trauma Guide. A source of evidence based treatment guidelines for dental trauma. http://www.dentaltraumaguide.org/Evidence_Based_Treatment.aspx.

213. The Dental Trauma Guide. History of the Dental Trauma Guide. http://www.dentaltraumaguide.org/History.aspx.

TOOTH SURVIVAL IN THE PERMANENT DENTITION

214. **Lauridsen E, Ahrensburg SS, Gerds TA, Hermann NV, Andreasen JO**. Crown fractures. Part 1. Healing complications of the pulp and PDL following crown fractures with or without concurrent luxation injury in permanent incisors. *Dent Traumatol* 2011;27: in preparation.

215. **Lauridsen E, Ahrensburg SS, Gerds TA, Hermann NV, Andreasen JO**. Crown fractures. Part 2. Prediction model for identification of high-risk patients after crown fracture in combination with concussion. *Dent Traumatol* 2011;27: in preparation.

216. **Lauridsen E, Ahrensburg SS, Gerds TA, Hermann NV, Andreasen JO**. Crown fractures. Part 3. Prediction model for identification of high-risk patients after crown fracture in combination with subluxation. *Dent Traumatol* 2011;27: in preparation.

217. **Lauridsen E, Ahrensburg SS, Gerds TA, Hermann NV, Andreasen JO**. Crown fractures. Part 4. Prediction model for identification of high-risk patients after crown fracture in combination with extrusion. *Dent Traumatol* 2011;27: in preparation.

218. **Lauridsen E, Ahrensburg SS, Gerds TA, Hermann NV, Andreasen JO**. Crown fractures. Part 5. Prediction model for identification of high-risk patients after crown fracture in combination with lateral luxation. *Dent Traumatol* 2011;27: in preparation.

219. **Lauridsen E, Ahrensburg SS, Gerds TA, Hermann NV, Andreasen JO**. Crown fractures. Part 6. Prediction model for identification of high-risk patients after crown fracture in combination with intrusion. *Dent Traumatol* 2011;27: in preparation.

220. **Andreasen JO, Bakland LK, Matras R, Andreasen FM**. Traumatic intrusion of permanent teeth. Part 2. A clinical study of the effect of preinjury and injury factors, such as sex, age, stage of root development, tooth location, and extent of injury including number of intruded teeth on 140 intruded permanent teeth. *Dent Traumatol* 2006;22:90–98.

221. **Andreasen JO, Bakland LK, Matras R, Andreasen FM**. Traumatic intrusion of permanent teeth. Part 3. A clinical study of the effect of treatment variables such as treatment delay, method of repositioning, type of splint, length of splinting and antibiotics on 140 teeth. *Dent Traumatol* 2006;22:99–111.

222. **Cvek M, Tsilingaridis G, Andreasen JO**. Survival of 534 incisors after intra-alveolar root fracture in patients aged 7–17 years. *Dent Traumatol* 2010;26: in press.

223. **Andreasen JO, Borum MK, Jacobsen HL, Andreasen FM**. Replantation of 400 avulsed permanent incisors. 1. Diagnosis of healing complications. *Endod Dent Traumatol* 1995; 11:51–58.

224. **Andreasen JO, Ahrensburg SS, Hillerup S, Kofod T, Schwartz O**. Healing complications following alveolar fractures in the permanent dentition. A clinical prospective study of 80 cases involving 194 teeth. *Dent Traumatol* 2011;27: in preparation.

INFORMATION FOR THE PATIENT ABOUT DENTAL TRAUMA

225. **Flores MT**. Information to the public, patients and emergency services on traumatic dental injuries. In: Andreasen JO, Andreasen FM, Andersson L (eds), *Textbook and Color Atlas of Traumatic Injuries to the Teeth* (4th edn). Oxford: Blackwell, Munksgaard 2007;35. pp. 869–875.

226. **Flores MT, Andersson L, Andreasen JO et al**. Guidelines for the management of traumatic dental injuries. I. Fractures and luxations of permanent teeth. *Dent Traumatol* 2007;23:66–71.

227. **Flores MT, Andersson L, Andreasen JO et al**. Guidelines for the management of traumatic dental injuries. II. Avulsion of permanent teeth *Dent Traumatol* 2007;23:130–136.

228. **Flores MT, Malmgren B, Andreasen JO et al**. Guidelines for the management of traumatic dental injuries. III. Primary teeth. *Dent Traumatol* 2007;23:196–202.

INFORMATION FOR THE PUBLIC ABOUT DENTAL TRAUMA

229. **Flores MT.** Information to the public, patients and emergency services on traumatic dental injuries. In: Andreasen JO, Andreasen FM, Andersson L (eds), *Textbook and Color Atlas of Traumatic Injuries to the Teeth* (4th edn). Oxford: Blackwell, Munksgaard, 2007. pp. 869–875.

230. **American Academy of Pediatric Dentistry**. Emergency Care 2009. http://www.aapd.org/publications/brochures/ecare.asp

231. **International Association of Paediatric Dentistry**. http://www.iapdworld.org/index.php?option=com_content&view=article&id=8&Itemid=19#12

232. **Flores MT, Malmgren B, Andreasen JO et al**. Guidelines for the management of traumatic dental injuries. III. Primary teeth. *Dent Traumatol* 2007;23:196–202.

233. **Yesil DZ, Gungor H**. Use of mouthguard rates among university athletes during sports activities in Erzurum, Turkey. *Dent Traumatol* 2009;25:318–322.

234. **Ma W**. Basketball players' experience of dental injury and awareness about mouthguards in China. *Dent Traumatol* 2008;24:430–434.

235. **Cohenca N, Roges RA, Roges R**. The incidence and severity of dental trauma in intercollegiate athletes. *J Am Dent Assoc* 2007;138:1121–1126.

236. **Lieger O, Graf C, El-Maaytah M, Von AT**. Impact of educational posters on the lay knowledge of school teachers regarding emergency management of dental injuries. *Dent Traumatol* 2009;25:406–412.

237. **McIntyre JD, Lee JY, Trope M, Vann WF, Jr**. Effectiveness of dental trauma education for elementary school staff. *Dent Traumatol* 2008;24:146–150.

238. **Al-Asfour A, Andersson L**. The effect of a leaflet given to parents for first aid measures after tooth avulsion. *Dent Traumatol* 2008;24:515–521.

239. **Al-Asfour A, Andersson L, Al-Jame Q**. School teachers' knowledge of tooth avulsion and dental first aid before and after receiving information about avulsed teeth and replantation. *Dent Traumatol* 2008;24:43–49.

240. **Tsukiboshi M**. *If You Know It, You Can Save the Tooth on Trauma*. Tokyo: Quintessence Publishing, 1996.

241. **Andreasen FM. O**. *Clast & the Bros. Blast*. Fribourg: Mediglobe, 1988.

242. **Levin L, Jeffet U, Zadik Y**. The effect of short term dental trauma lecture on knowledge of high-risk population: an intervention study of 336 young adults. *Dent Traumatol* 2010;26:86–9.

243. **de Vasconcellos LG, Brentel AS, Vanderlei AD, de Vasconcellos LM, Valera MC, de Araújo MA**. Knowledge of general dentists in the current guidelines for emergency treatment of avulsed teeth and dental trauma prevention. *Dental Traumatol* 2009;25:578–83. Epub 2009 Sep 24.

244. **International Association of Dental Traumatology**. http://www.iadt-dentaltrauma.org/web/index.php?option=com_content&task=section&id=6&Itemid=29

245. **Glendor U**. Has the education of professional caregivers and lay people in dental trauma care failed? *Dent Traumatol* 2009;25:12–18.

246. **Addo ME, Parekh S, Moles DR, Roberts GJ**. Knowledge of dental trauma first aid (DTFA): the example of avulsed incisors casualty departments and schools in London. *Br Dent J* 2007;202:E27.

247. **Feldens EG, Feldens CA, Kramer PF, da Silva KG, Munari CC, Brei VA**. Understanding school teacher's knowledge regarding dental trauma: a basis for future interventions. *Dent Traumatol* 2010;26:158–63. Epub 2010 Jan 19.

248. **Andreasen JO, Lauridsen E, Christensen SS**. Development of an interactive dental trauma guide. *Pediatr Dent* 2009;31:133–136.

PREVENTION OF TRAUMATIC DENTAL INJURIES

249. **Sigurdsson A**. Prevention of dental and oral injuries. In: Andreasen JO, Andreasen FM, Andersson L (eds), *Textbook and Color Atlas of Traumatic Injuries to the Teeth* (4th edn). Oxford: Blackwell, Munksgaard, 2007. pp. 869–875.

250. **Benson BW, Mohatadi NG, Rose MS, Meeuwisse WH**. Head and neck injuries among ice hockey players wearing full face shields vs half face shields. *J Am Med Assoc* 1999;282:2328–2332.

251. **Wisniewski JF, Guskiewica K, Trope M, Sigurdsson A**. Incidence of cerebral concussions associated with type of mouthguard used in college football. *Dent Traumatol* 2004;20:143–149.

252. **Stuart MJ, Smith AM, Malo-Ortiguera SA, Fischer TL, Larson DR**. A comparison of facial protection and the incidence of head, neck, and facial injuries in Junior A hockey players. A function of individual playing time. *Am J Sports Med* 2002;30:39–44.

253. **Yamada T, Sawaki Y, Tomida S, Tohnai I, Ueda M**. Oral injury and mouthguard usage by athletes in Japan. *Endod Dent Traumatol* 1998;14:84–87.

254. **Kvittem B, Hardie NA, Roettger M, Conry J**. Incidence of orofacial injuries in high school sports. *J Public Health Dent* 1998;58:288–293.

255. **Castaldi CL**. Mouthguards in contact sports. *J Connecticut State Dent Assoc* 1974;48:233–241.

256. **Hayrinen-Immonen R, Sane J, Perkki K, Malmstrom M**. A six-year follow-up study of sports-related dental injuries in children and adolescents. *Endod Dent Traumatol* 1990;6:208–212.

257. **Hendrick K, Farrelly P, Jagger R**. Oro-facial injuries and mouthguard use in elite female field hockey players. *Dent Traumatol* 2008;24:189–192.

258. **Ma W**. Basketball players' experience of dental injury and awareness about mouthguard in China. *Dent Traumatol* 2008;24:430–434.

259. **Knapik JJ, Marshall SW, Lee RB, Darakjy SS, Jones SB, Mitchener TA, delaCruz GG, Jones BH**. Mouthguards in sport activities: history, physical properties and injury prevention effectiveness. *Sports Med* 2007;37:117–144.

260. **ADA Council on Access, Prevention and Interprofessional Relations; ADA Council on Scientific Affairs**. Using mouthguards to reduce the incidence and severity of sports-related oral injuries. *J Am Dent Assoc* 2006;137:1712–20;quiz 1731. Summary for patients in: *J Am Dent Assoc* 2006;137:1772.

261. **Johnston T, Messer LB**. An in vitro study of the efficacy of mouthguard protection for dentoalveolar injuries in deciduous and mixed dentitions. *Endod Dent Traumatol* 1996;12:277–285.

262. **Hoffmann J, Alfter G, Rudolph NK, Goz G**. Experimental comparative study of various mouthguards. *Endod Dent Traumatol* 1999;15:157–163.

263. **Takeda T, Ishigami K, Nakajima K, Naitoh K, Kurokawa K, Handa J, Shomura M, Regner CW**. Are all mouthguards the same and safe to use? Part 2. The influence of anterior occlusion against a direct impact on maxillary incisors. *Dent Traumatol* 2008 ;24:360–365.

264. **Takeda T, Ishigami K, Ogawa T, Nakajima K, Shibusawa M, Shimada A, Regner CW**. Are all mouthguards the same and safe to use? The influence of occlusal supporting mouthguards in decreasing bone distortion and fractures. *Dent Traumatol* 2004;20:150–156.

265. **McNutt T, Shannon SW, Wright JT, Feistein RA**. Oral trauma in adolescent athletes: a study of mouthguards. *Pediatric Dentistry* 1989;11:205–213.

266. **Nysether S**. Dental injuries among Norwegian soccer players. *Community Dent Oral Epidemiol* 1987;15:141–143.

267. **Oikarinen KS, Salonen MA**. Introduction to four custom-made mouth protectors constructed of single and double layers for activists in contact sports. *Endod Dent Traumatol* 1993;9:19–24.

268. **Zadik Y, Levin L**. Does a free-of-charge distribution of boil-and-bite mouthguards to young adult amateur sportsmen affect oral and facial trauma? *Dent Traumatol* 2009;25:69–72.

269. **Patrick DG, van Noort R, Found MS**. Scale of protection and the various types of sports mouthguard. *Br J Sports Med* 2005;39:278–281.

270. **Truman BI, Gooch BF, Sulemana I, Gift HC, Horowitz AM, Evans CA, et al.** Reviews of evidence on interventions to prevent dental caries, oral and pharyngeal cancers, and sports-related craniofacial injuries. *Am J Prev Med* 2002;23:21–54.

271. **Roberts JE**. *Wisconsin Interscholastic Athletic Association 1970 Benefit Plan Summary*. Supplement to the 47th Official Handbook of the Wisconsin Interscholastic Athletic Association 1970:1–77.

272. **Sane J**. Comparison of maxillofacial and dental injuries in four contact team sports: American football, bandy, basketball, and handball. *Am J Sports Med* 1988;16:647–651.

273. **Lieger O, von Arx T**. Orofacial/cerebral injuries and the use of mouthguards by professional athletes in Switzerland. *Dent Traumatol* 2006;22:1–6.

274. **Maestrello-de Moya MG, Primosch RE**. Orofacial trauma and mouth-protector wear among high school varsity basketball players. *ASDC J Dent Child* 1989;56:36–39.

275. **Labella CR, Smith BW, Sigurdsson A**. Effect of mouthguards on dental injuries and concussions in college basketball. *Med Sci Sports Exerc* 2002;34:41–44.

276. **de Cardenas SO**. Mouth protectors during the 1st World Amateur Boxing Championship. *Rev Cubana Estomatol* 1975;12:49–66.

277. **Vulcan AP, Cameron MH, Watson WL**. Mandatory bicycle helmet use: experience in Victoria, Australia. *World J Surg* 1992;16:389–397.

278. **Acton CH, Nixon JW, Clark RC**. Bicycle riding and oral/maxillofacial trauma in young children. *Med J Aust* 1996;165:249–251.

279. **Linn S, Smith D, Sheps S**. Epidemiology of bicycle injury, head injury and helmet use among children in British Colombia: a five year descriptive study. Canadian hospitals injury reporting and prevention program (CHIRPP). *Inj Prev* 1998;4:122–125.

280. **Thompson DC, Nunn MF, Thompson RS, Rivara FP**. Effectiveness of bicycle safety helmets in preventing serious facial injury. *J Am Med Ass* 1997;276:1774–1775.

281. **Müller KE, Persic R, Pohl Y, Krastl G, Filippi A**. Dental injuries in mountain biking – a survey in Switzerland, Austria, Germany and Italy. *Dent Traumatol* 2008;24:522–527.

282. **Kelly P, Sanson T, Strange G, Orsay E**. A prospective study of the impact of helmet usage on motorcycle trauma. *Ann Emerg Med* 1991;20: 852–856.

283. **Bachulis BL, Sanster W, Gorrell GW, et al**. Patterns of injury in helmet and nonhelmet motorcyclists. *Am J Surg* 1988;155:708–711.

284. **Reath DB, Kirby J, Lynch M, Maull KI**. Patterns of maxillofacial injuries in restrained and unrestrained motor vehicle crash victims. *J Trauma* 1989;29:806–809.

Index

Traumatic Dental Injuries: A Manual, Third Edition   © J.O. Andreasen, L.K. Bakland, M.T. Flores, F.M. Andreasen and L. Andersson
Published 2011 by Blackwell Publishing Ltd